Laboratory Animal Law: Legal Control of the Use of Animals in Research

Second Edition

Kevin Dolan

SThL(JusCan), BD, DipLaw, FIAT

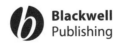

Blackwell
Publishing

Blackwell Publishing editorial offices:
Blackwell Publishing Ltd, 9600 Garsington Road, Oxford OX4 2DQ, UK
  Tel: +44 (0)1865 776868
Blackwell Publishing Professional, 2121 State Avenue, Ames, Iowa 50014-8300, USA
  Tel: +1 515 292 0140
Blackwell Publishing Asia Pty Ltd, 550 Swanston Street, Carlton, Victoria 3053, Australia
  Tel: +61 (0)3 8359 1011

First edition published 2000 by Blackwell Science Ltd
Second edition published 2007 by Blackwell Publishing Ltd

ISBN: 978-1-4051-6282-1

Library of Congress Cataloging-in-Publication Data
Dolan, Kevin.
    Laboratory animal law : legal control of the use of animals in
research / Kevin Dolan. — 2nd ed.
        p. ; cm.
    Includes bibliographical references and index.
    ISBN: 978-1-4051-6282-1 (pbk. : alk. paper)
    1. Laboratory animals—Law and legislation—Great Britain.   2. Animal
experimentation—Law and legislation—Great Britain. I. Title.
    [DNLM: 1. Animal Experimentation—legislation & jurisprudence—Great
Britain. 2. Animals, Laboratory—Great Britain. QY 33 FA1 D659L 2007]
    KD3426.D65 2007
    344.4104′9—dc22
                                                        2006035498

A catalogue record for this title is available from the British Library

Set in 11/13 pt Bembo
by Graphicraft Limited, Hong Kong
Printed and bound in Singapore
by Fabulous Printers Pte Ltd

For further information on Blackwell Publishing, visit our website:
www.blackwellpublishing.com

Contents

Preface

This book, *Laboratory Animal Law: Legal Control of the Use of Animals in Research*, is intended to replace my previous work on this topic, *Laboratory Animal Law* (2000). This is not merely a second edition of the previous book on the Animals (Scientific Procedures) Act 1986 [A(SP)A]. The A(SP)A has not changed in the intervening six years, but the impact of the Home Office (HO) on the administration of the Act has increased as the years have rolled by since 1986. The influence in practice of the Inspectorate needs to be more and more taken into consideration if one is to properly understand the legal control of the use of animals in research in practice, at the level of the animal facility or in the implementation of the project licence.

The welfare of laboratory animals is demanded by legislation and is, I hope, adequately dealt with in the text. This is by no means intended to be a treatise on animal law in general. It has been written primarily for the use of those involved in animal studies, especially those concerned with animals in research. It is hoped that it will give them an overall view of their legal obligations towards the animals in their care. The public I have in mind is based on the numerous and various animal technicians who have faced me in class during a period of more than 20 years. If the tone, therefore, tends to be lay rather than legal, it will show that I have learnt more from them, perhaps, than they from me. I am fully aware that the material in this book is available elsewhere, particularly on the internet. This text is intended to provide a useful compilation of legal material of interest to busy, non-legal-minded scientists and technicians in research using animals and may be of value to concerned members of the public.

The main emphasis in the text will obviously be on the Animals (Scientific Procedures) Act 1986 (referred to throughout the text as the A(SP)A). Other legislation, such as the Animal Welfare Act, the Veterinary Surgeons Act 1966, the Agriculture (Miscellaneous Provisions) Act 1968, the Animal Health Act 1981 and the European Directive 86/609/EEC, will be commented upon in so far as they may be relevant to laboratory animals. The impact of European law on this area of legislation will be noted. Passing reference will be made to some animal laws, such as the Wildlife and Countryside Act 1981, which are peripheral to the main theme of the book.

Numerous Statutory Instruments, both Orders and Regulations, along with Directives, Codes of Practice, Guidelines and the Stipulations of Good Laboratory Practice bearing on animal experimentation could be of interest to many scientists and technicians dealing with animals and are often very relevant to their particular area of work. Unfortunately both space and time are limited. Where appropriate I will refer to such documents and attempt to indicate the best place to find them, particularly on websites. There is a list of relevant websites at the end of the text.

In such specialised areas there is the obvious need to consult the actual documents themselves. Their details would be difficult to paraphrase in a work such as this. Furthermore, it must be stressed that where there are actual legal problems or disputes of a litigious nature, the appropriate legal experts must be consulted if an authoritative solution is being sought.

Kevin Dolan

Acknowledgements

The order in which the material is presented corresponds with my own past lectures aligned to the Institute of Animal Technology's syllabus for the Fellowship Examination. Gratitude for the moulding of this text is due to the many students who listened patiently and sometimes spurred me on. Joanna Cruden, Steve Cubit, Lorraine Gagen, Jessica Gruninger and Jackie Taylor spring readily to mind. Thank you also to those who have encouraged me along the way. Steve Barnet, Pilar Browne, John Gregory, Janice Lobb, Peter McLoughlin and Ron Raymond certainly fall into this category.

As a member of both the IAT and the LASA, I have drawn copiously from the periodicals and publications emanating from those informative and prolific sources of relevant material. I was particularly grateful to Phil Ruddock, editor of the IAT Bulletin, for up-to-date material.

The Research Defence Society generously made available to me a large amount of useful source material, which I would like to acknowledge with gratitude. The Society stands out as a positive, outspoken force in the controversy surrounding biological research.

Without fruitful consultation with the Home Office Inspectorate, along with their ready supply of relevant material, this book would not have been possible. The material taken from the Home Office Guidance Notes and from some DEFRA publications is Crown copyright and reproduced with permission of the Controller of Her Majesty's Stationery Office. DEFRA's material, particularly the website, proved a useful source for material especially in Chapters 18 to 22.

Special acknowledgements must be paid to those friends who collaborated with me in the production of this text. New material on animal welfare and the import and export of animals was contributed by Jas Barley. New material on the role of the NACWO and the codes of practice was contributed by Tim Betts. New material on drugs in research was contributed by Pat Coulson. New material on the NVS and Veterinary Surgeons Act was contributed by Fraser Darling. New material on animal transport was contributed by Roger Francis. The secretarial burden was ably shouldered and skilfully manipulated on her computer by Lerena Dyer with the able assistance of Lovern Dyer. I was helped in my own IT ventures in the writing of the book by Pat Barker. Thank you one and all.

Abbreviations

APC	Animals Procedure Committee
A(SP)A	Animals (Scientific Procedures) Act 1986
BUAV	British Union for the Abolition of Vivisection
CD	Certificate of Designation
CH	Certificate Holder
CITES	Convention on International Trade in Endangered Species
COSHH	Control of Substances Hazardous to Health
DE	Designated Establishment
DEFRA	Department for the Environment, Food and Rural Affairs
ECVAM	European Centre for the Validation of Alternative Methods
GLP	Good Laboratory Practice
GUIDANCE	Home Office Guidance (on the operation of the A(SP)A)
HO	Home Office
HOI	Home Office Inspector
IAT	Institute of Animal Technology
LASA	Laboratory Animal Science Association
LAVA	Laboratory Animal Veterinary Association
LERP or ERP	Local Ethical Review Process
MAFF	Ministry of Agriculture, Fisheries and Food (cf. DEFRA)
NACWO	Named Animal Care and Welfare Officer
NAVS	National Anti-vivisection Society
NVS	Named Veterinary Surgeon
OJ	Official Journal of the European Community
PCD	Home Office Documents to Certificate Holders
PIL	Personal Licence
PODE	Place other than a Designated Establishment
PPL	Project Licence
RIDDOR	Reporting of Injuries, Diseases and Dangerous Occurrences Regulations
SI	Statutory Instrument
SOP	Standing Operating Procedure
RDS	Research Defence Society
3Rs	Replacement, Reduction and Refinement
UFAW	Universities Federation for Animal Welfare

The acronym MAFF featured frequently in the first edition. It should be noted that the Department for Environment, Food and Rural Affairs (DEFRA) was created in June 2001 from the Ministry of Agriculture, Fisheries and Food and from the environmental and countryside business areas of the then Department of the Environment, Transport and the Regions. It has not always been therefore a simple case of substituting DEFRA for MAFF or DETR. Some material used comes from the past, is still valid, and drew its legal support from MAFF or DETR. Thus in some circumstances one of those acronyms is an appropriate reference and may still occur. (cf. http://www.defra.gov.uk/corporate/index.asp).

In connection with some of the above arcane terms, I think that an anticipatory apology may not be out of place. In any subject, but particularly in law, there is a tendency to become immersed in the associated jargon. Often we are so familiar with our own technical expressions, whose meanings seem so obvious to ourselves, that we tend to forget that to the outsider they may have an air of mystery about them.

This was brought home to me after lecturing for four hours on the A(SP)A. A Swiss scientist in Oxford expressed her appreciation of the instructive session. She ensured me that she had understood all that was said except one recurring phrase: 'Home Office'. She knew what 'home' meant and what 'office' meant. She could not comprehend what was the relevance of either term to laboratory animals. The fact that the title of Secretary of State applies to politicians as diverse as a Foreign Minister and the member of the government responsible for Northern Ireland, confused the matter further. In this book 'Secretary of State' refers to one of Her Majesty's Principal Secretaries of State, 'Secretary of State for the Home Department', popularly known as the Home Secretary. At the time of writing (2006) he is the Rt. Hon. John Reid. 'Home Office' is the familiar title of the part of government that deals with the various internal affairs of our nation.

Part I

Introduction

Chapter 1

The Legal Protection of Animals

The growth of legislation

The main pieces of legislation protecting animals in the UK have been the Protection of Animals Act 1911 and in Scotland the Protection of Animals Act 1912. Most legal cases involving animals are prosecuted under one or other of these Acts. Unlike the Animals (Scientific Procedures) Act 1986, the 1911 Act allowed for the process of private prosecution. This rendered it a useful instrument for bodies actively involved in combating animal cruelty. However, it was not until the twentieth century that such a comprehensive piece of animal protection legislation evolved. The first animal protection Act was of limited application – the Martin's Act 1822. Richard Martin, a barrister and MP for Galway, was, with William Wilberforce, one of the founding fathers in 1824 of the Society for the Prevention of Cruelty to Animals, which later blossomed into the RSPCA. Although Martin's Act was entitled 'an Act to prevent the cruel and improper Treatment of Cattle', its scope was somewhat wider than just the protection of cattle as the term is now generally understood, as the full text of the Act implies.

> 'Whereas it is expedient to prevent the cruel and improper Treatment of Horses, Mares, Geldings, Mules, Asses, Cows, Heifers, Steers, Oxen, Sheep and other Cattle: May it therefore please your majesty that it may be enacted; . . . and if the Party or Parties accused shall be convicted of any such offence . . . he, she or they so convicted shall forfeit and pay any Sum not exceeding Five Pounds nor less than Ten Shillings.'

By the time we come to 1911, such misdemeanours were viewed far more gravely and hard labour was included among the possible penalties which could be imposed on offenders. Modern sanctions under the 1911 Act are not so draconian. The numerous amendments, in which the 1911 Act abounds, moderated the penalties as well as introducing other features into the legal prevention of cruelty to animals. The penalties usually appear to be short terms of imprisonment, moderate fines or community service. A more recent amendment, the Protection of Animals (Amendment) Act 1988, did, however, increase the powers of the courts to deal with offenders in this area. It enabled the court to disqualify a person from having custody of an animal on a first conviction of cruelty and increased the penalties relating to animal fights. It made further provision with respect to attendance at such fights in England and Wales, and penalised attendance at such fights in Scotland.

The range of animals originally brought within the protection of Martin's Act was gradually extended. The Cruelty to Animals Acts of 1835 and 1849 proved to be wider in their application. It appears that around the 1850s an enterprising lawyer was able to harness the breadth of this legislation to prosecute a person suspected of cruelty to some children. He used this approach as there was no specific legal protection of them at the time. Limited though Martin's Act was, a case under it brought by the RSPCA was instrumental in the success in the campaign to pass the Cruelty to Animals Act 1876 (the predecessor of the Animals (Scientific Procedures) Act). Dr Magnan, a Frenchman, demonstrated at a public meeting of the BMA in 1874 that while injection of alcohol produced anaesthesia in a dog, absinthe caused convulsions. He wished to draw attention to the dangers of absinthe. Dr Magnan had left the country before the prosecution was effective.

'Animal' in the 1911 Act

Within the 1911 Act the term 'animal' was not extended to all animals, just as in the Cruelty to Animals Act 1876, where the term 'animal' was intended to cover no more than vertebrates. Qualification for protection under the 1911 Act was restricted to domestic or captive animals.

Under s. 15 'domestic' includes animals commonly considered domesticated, such as horses, cattle, cats, dogs and birds as well as any other species which has been 'sufficiently tamed to serve some purpose for the use of man'.

The term 'captive' covers any other species, including any bird, fish or reptile, which is in captivity or under some form of control (such as caging or pinioning) to keep it confined. The captivity must be something more than temporary prevention from escape or inability (not caused by man) to escape. The precise meaning of the term 'captive' has been defined by case law. Unlike the 1876 and the 1986 Acts concerned with animals in research, the 1911 Act has produced abundant and fruitful precedents for the development of reliable case law.

The 1911 Act and the A(SP)A

Between 1986 and 1999 there have been four prosecutions involving animals used in research. Only two of these were under the A(SP)A and are noted in the appropriate place. Even so, in the second case (*Lord Advocate* v. *Bairden*, July 1998) there had been offences charged under the (Scotland) Protection of Animals 1912 Act for which a plea of not guilty was accepted.

The first case between 1986 and 1999 involving laboratory animals was a prosecution, but not under the A(SP)A, of a company and one of its directors in 1989.

They were found guilty of offences following an incident in which 79 beagles died en route by ferry to Sweden. The incident did not come directly within the scope of A(SP)A because it had occurred before s. 7 (apropos Schedule 2) had come into force. The second case, brought under the 1911 Act, was against two animal technicians for causing dogs unnecessary suffering. It was first heard in Huntingdon on 7 June 1997 and resulted in their conviction. The evidence in the case came from a Channel 4 TV programme on 26 March 1997 entitled 'It's a Dog's Life' in the *Countryside Undercover* series (APC Report, 1997). These cases will be referred to later in the chapter on prosecutions.

The need to take notice of the relevance of other legislation apart from the A(SP)A in the setting of animal units was highlighted by a case commenced in Bromley magistrates' court and completed in Croydon Crown court. In *British Union for the Abolition of Vivisection* v. *Royal College of Surgeons* (1985), the RCS was unsuccessfully prosecuted by the BUAV under the 1911 Act. The BUAV had accused the RCS of neglect of a female monkey in unsuitable environmental conditions as regards temperature, and claimed that as a result of this negligence the animal had sustained an injury and had suffered unnecessarily.

Further comments on the 1911 Act

With the enactment of the Animal Welfare Act (2006), what has been said about the Protection of Animals Act 1911 may be merely of historical interest. The nature and impact of the new Act will be commented upon in Chapter 20.

According to the Animal Welfare Act the major portion of the 1911 Act is repealed by the enactment of this bill – ss. 1 to 7 and ss. 9 to 13, parts of ss. 14 and 15. The remaining parts of the 1911 Act not affected by this repeal are as follows:

- S. 8 is concerned with the selling, using, etc. of poisoned grain.
- Part of s. 14 is concerned with appeals against conviction.
- S. 15(b) is concerned with the definition of 'domestic animal', which means any horse, ass, mule, bull, sheep, pig, goat, dog, cat, fowl or any other animal of whatsoever kind or species and whether a quadruped or not, which has been or is being sufficiently tamed to serve some purpose for the use of man.
- S. 15(d) expands on the definition of the 'domestic animals' mentioned in s. 15(b), for example, fowl includes swans and pigeons.
- Ss. 16 to 19 are of little consequence and would appear to be already redundant. They deal with the application of the 1911 Act to Ireland but not to Scotland, and other legally technical details.
- Schedule 1 is concerned with knackers.
- Schedule 2 repeals some previous animal legislation.

Some of the above topics would have already been absorbed into past legislation.

The use of anaesthetics on animals

The Protection of Animals (Anaesthetics) Act 1954 was amended in certain matters by the Protection of Animals (Anaesthetics) Act 1964. For easier understanding of the legal position, I think it is preferable to present the final result of the fusing of the 1964 amendments with the original 1954 Act.

The principle on which the legislation is based is that any operation involving interference with sensitive tissues or the bone structure of an animal without a properly administered anaesthetic shall be deemed to be performed without 'due care and humanity'. The provision does not apply to injections or extractions using a hollow needle nor to operations listed in Schedule 1 of the 1954 Act. The variations introduced in 1964 revoked or qualified aspects of this Schedule. The present exceptions, when anaesthetics need not be used on an animal, are:

(1)   *Regulated procedures* in which the use of anaesthetics is not required under the authority of the A(SP)A. One must always be aware, however, of Schedule 2A of the A(SP)A.
(2)   Emergency first aid to save life or relieve pain.
(3)   Docking of the tail of a dog before its eyes are open. Since July 1994 this operation can legally only be done by a veterinary surgeon but the Royal College of Veterinary Surgeons in 1974 had declared the practice unethical. Such an operation, therefore, would need to be justified in relation to the well-being of the puppy.
(4)   Amputation of the dew-claws of a dog before its eyes are open.
(5)   The provisions as regards castration of equidae were revoked by the 1964 amendment and are now redundant.
(6)   Minor operations by a veterinary surgeon, which because of their quickness or painlessness are customarily so performed without an anaesthetic.
(7)   Minor procedures which would not customarily be performed by a veterinary surgeon. These could include some procedures on agricultural animals.

The 1964 amendment stressed that castration, dehorning and debudding are not to be regarded *per se* as 'minor operations' or 'minor procedures' (as in (6) and (7) above). The 1964 amendment specifically ruled out castration by the use of any device constricting the flow of blood to the scrotum unless applied within the first week of life. The amendment also ruled out the dehorning of cattle or the disbudding of calves without an anaesthetic, except by chemical cauterisation applied in the first week of life.

As regards other procedures on agricultural animals, lambs' tails can only be docked by a device constricting blood flow to the tail if this is applied within the first week of life. According to the Docking and Nicking of Horses Act 1949, such a practice with respect to a horse, pony, mule or hinny was forbidden unless certified as necessary by a veterinary surgeon. (Hardly relevant here, but it would be a pity to omit such a little statutory rustic gem.)

Deer antlers in velvet must be removed under anaesthetic sufficient to prevent pain unless done in an emergency or authorised under the A(SP)A (Removal of Antlers in Velvet (Anaesthetics) Order 1980).

Neither the 1954 Act nor the 1964 Amendment apply to 'fowl or other bird, fish or reptile'. Failure to use anaesthesia for an operation on a bird, a fish or a reptile would not automatically imply in law that an operation had been carried out without 'due care and humanity'.

The effect of the Animal Welfare Act (2006) on these Anaesthetics Acts will be negligible. It is proposed that only s. 2(2) of the 1954 Act and s. 2(1)(a) of the 1964 Act be repealed. This means that neither Act should be cited in future as Protection of Animals Acts.

Part II

The Animals (Scientific Procedures) Act 1986 – A(SP)A

Chapter 2

The Coming of the Law on Laboratory Animals

The Cruelty to Animals Act 1876

When in 1809 Lord Erskine introduced a bill into the House of Lords concerned with the use of animals in research, he was regarded as eccentric and his suggested legislation was summarily dismissed as hardly worthy of serious consideration. Society at that time openly condoned cock-fighting and bear-baiting.

During the nineteenth century, however, there was a gradual build-up of demands for legislation to protect animals used in research. The Society for the Prevention of Cruelty to Animals had been founded in 1824 and by the 1880s the Anti-Vivisection Society had been established. There were already strong feelings in high places on the matter as instanced by Disraeli's correspondence with Queen Victoria. Leading scientists were also concerned. A petition signed by Huxley, Jenner, Owen, the Presidents of the Royal College of Physicians and Surgeons and other eminent scientists including Darwin called for the control of animal experimentation.

A Royal Commission was set up in 1875 which ushered in the Cruelty to Animals Act 1876. This Act, the first of its kind in the world, controlled 'painful experiments' on animals for specific purposes and under certain conditions. This Act was a great leap forward in concern for animals. It was, however, far from perfect; after all, it was a 'first off'. Its use of the crucial phrase 'painful experiments' in an exclusive sense implied that some uses of animals in research that could be disturbing were, as the lawyers would say 'outwith' the Act. Strictly speaking, the term 'experiment', by definition, could only include procedures by which new knowledge could be gained. Thus such practices as passaging tumours or the production of antibodies could be considered as outside the reach of the legislation. Furthermore, the term 'painful' could not literally include experiments or other uses of animals in research that could give rise to great discomfort, short of pain as such. The confusion caused by these inadequacies in the legislative drafting of the 1876 Act were obviated by the skilful drafting (under the guidance of the then Home Office Minister, David Mellor) of the 1986 Act. The inapt phrase 'painful experiment' was replaced in s. 2(1) of the 1986 Act by the crucial and more explicit term 'a regulated procedure'.

> '. . . any experimental or other scientific procedure applied to a protected animal which may have the effect of causing that animal pain, suffering, distress or lasting harm.'

On account of the aforementioned deficiencies in the 1876 Act and continual and forceful agitation from pressure groups, an abortive attempt was made to produce consensus on the reform of the 1876 Act. A Departmental Committee on Experiments on Animals was set up, which produced in 1965 the Littlewood Report. This was a lengthy and informative report, but unfortunately it was of little lasting consequence.

The use of animals under the 1876 Act rose steadily during the twentieth century, reaching by 1973 the significant figure of 5.5 million per annum. This high number sparked off further controversy and caused some interested parties to call into question the ability of the 1876 Act to control animal experimentation.

At a deeper level than existing legislation, debate was provoked on the topic of ethical justification for the use of animals in research. Attitudes hardened, opinions crystallised and the various pressure groups intensified their activities. The lobbyists of various societies instigated numerous attempts to produce new, usually stricter, legislation on animal experimentation by means of private Members' bills throughout the 1970s.

In 1978 a Council of Europe Committee of experts started work on a draft convention for the protection of animals used for experimental and other scientific purposes. In 1980 the then Home Secretary invited his Advisory Committee on Animal Experiments to discuss framework legislation to replace the 1876 Act. In March 1986 the Council of Europe's Convention for the Protection of Vertebrate Animals used for Experimental and other Scientific Procedures was promulgated. In the UK a comprehensive supplementary White Paper to a previous 1983 White Paper on the subject had already been issued with serious intent in May 1985. The 1985 White Paper was given legislative form in keeping with the European Convention as the Animals (Scientific Procedures) Act 1986 (A(SP)A).

The European Convention had been adopted by the Council of Europe (a supra-national body distinct from the EEC) in May 1985, opened for signatures on 18 March 1986, and had received sufficient signatures of Member States (including the UK) to bring the Convention into force on 1 October 1986 prior to ratification by individual nations. Even by 2000, ratification had not been forthcoming from all the signatories. The presence or absence of formal ratification is no reflection on the sincerity with which the provisions of the Convention have been applied in practice. The then EEC (now the EU) legislated for Member States. Directive 86/609/EEC demanded compliance with the Convention within three years from 1986. Up to the present (2007), application of the stipulations of the Convention have varied even within the EU.

The 1876 Act: a valediction

Before passing on to deal in detail with the consequence of the European Convention that is our own A(SP)A, it may not be out of place to refer to the worth of the Cruelty to Animals Act 1876. Inadequate though it may have been, it was a unique legal phenomenon, worldwide, certainly for nearly 50 years. Apart from in Germany and Italy, it was not matched outside the British legal system for over a century (see *Ethics, Animals and Science*, K. Dolan, Blackwell Science, Oxford, 1999). In spite of its many critics, the 1876 Act weathered the storms for over a century and did not lack effectiveness. In spite of rumours to the contrary, there were in fact three prosecutions under this Act.

In 1876, Dr Arbrath was prosecuted for advertising – obviously a case of public display – a lecture on poisons in which experiments would be shown. The advertisement appeared three days after the Act was passed. Although no experiment was actually performed, there was a conviction with a nominal fine. Dr Arbrath belonged to the local SPCA (a plebeian form no doubt of the RSPCA), who had refused to prosecute him (*BMJ* 1876 (ii) 545).

In 1881, Dr David Ferrier was prosecuted by the Victoria Street Society (precursor of the NAVS) for performing experiments on the brain. The prosecution failed because the operations were actually performed by a Dr G. F. Yeo, who held the required licence and certificates (*BMJ* 1881 (ii) 836–42).

In 1913 Dr Warrington Yorke was prosecuted for cruelty to a donkey involving a drug possibly useful against sleeping sickness, which produces a species of paralysis. The prosecution failed. Dr Yorke was properly licensed and the court decided that the suffering involved was not unnecessary (*Times Law Reports*, 29 May 1914).

A peculiar case prior to the 1876 Act ushered in the passing of the Act. In 1874, a Frenchman, Dr Magnan demonstrated at a public meeting of the BMA that while an injection of alcohol produced anaesthesia in a dog, an injection of absinthe caused convulsions. Although this procedure was done for the best of motives, to show the dangers of absinthe, an attempt was made to prosecute him under Martin's Act 1822. By the time the prosecution had got under way, Dr Magnan had left the country. It is difficult to understand why the prosecution was under Martin's Act, which was primarily concerned with cattle (*cf. Valiant Crusade*, A. W. Moss, Cassell, London, 1961, pp. 77–8).

The 1876 Act was not completely relegated to the realms of history. Its title lives on in the legislation of the Irish Republic. New legislation on the use of animals in research was brought into force by the Irish Statutory Instruments (SI No. 566), European Communities (Amendment of Cruelty to Animals Act 1876) Regulations 2002. It was issued by the Minister of Health and Children, Michael Martin on 5 December 2002. This amended form of the Cruelty to Animals Act 1876 is a legislative entwining of the 1876 Act and European Directive No. 86/609/EEC.

Scope of the Animals (Scientific Procedures) Act 1986

The scope of this Act was clearly set out in the 1991 Report (p. 22) of the Animal Procedures Committee:

> '8.2 The Act provides for the licensing of experimental and other scientific procedures carried out on protected animals, which may cause pain, suffering,

distress or lasting harm. Such work is referred to in the Act as a regulated procedure. This means that the Act controls the whole range of scientific procedures, from major surgery to the many thousands of scientific procedures which are so minor that they do not require anaesthesia, like the taking of a blood sample.

8.3 Protected animals are defined in the Act as all living vertebrate animals [and *Octopus vulgaris* since 1993] except man and the definition extends to foetal, larval or embryonic forms which have reached specified stages in their development. Under the Act an animal is regarded as "living" until the permanent cessation of circulation or complete destruction of its brain. It follows that procedures carried out on decerebrate animals are subject to the controls of the Act.

8.4 The Act extended controls to some scientific work not covered by earlier legislation. Such work includes, in particular, some breeding animals with genetic defects; production of antisera and other blood products; the maintenance and passage of tumours and parasites; and the administration for a scientific purpose of an anaesthetic, analgesic, tranquiliser or other drug to dull perception. The humane killing of an animal for scientific purposes requires licence authority in certain circumstances.

8.5 The controls do not extend to procedures applied to animals in the course of recognised veterinary, agricultural or animal husbandry practice, procedures for identification of animals for scientific purposes, if this causes no more than momentary pain or distress and no lasting harm; or clinical tests on animals for evaluating a veterinary product under authority of an Animal Test Certificate under the Medicines Act 1968.'

Further details of how the scope of this Act is expressed in practice are to be found in the Guidance on the Operation of the Animals (Scientific Procedures) Act 1986, as amended in 2000. As this document is commonly referred to as the Home Office Guidance, it will be referred to in this text as the Guidance. Further details of changes as regards the administration of A(SP)A appear in Home Office communications.

Sections of A(SP)A

Each section of the Act is concerned with a specific area of the legislation on the use of animals in research. These are outlined in Table 2.1. Many of these amendments appeared in 1998 and will be dealt with later when appropriate.

An enabling Act

The adaptability of the 1986 Act arises from the fact that it is an enabling Act. By the power of enabling, indicated within the Act itself, the appropriate minister, in

Table 2.1 Sections of the 1986 Act concerned with specific areas of the legislation on the use of animals in research

Section	Area of legislation covered
s. 1	defines 'Protected Animal'. (A)
s. 2	defines a 'Regulated Procedure'.
s. 3	outlines the nature of a personal licence in the setting of a project licence and specified place.
s. 4	gives details on the granting of a personal licence. (A)
s. 5	describes in detail the nature of a project licence. (A)
s. 6	deals with Designated Scientific Procedure Establishments, mentioning the NACWO (was 'person in day to day care') and the NVS.
s. 7	deals with Designated Breeding and Supplying Establishments. (A)
s. 8	calls for the paying of the fees by the CH.
s. 9	refers to those who may be consulted by the Secretary of State.
s. 10	refers to the conditions on licences and certificates. (A)
s. 11	is concerned with the variation or revocation of licences or certificates.
s. 12	outlines the process of making representation against an adverse verdict from the Secretary of State.
s. 13	allows for suspension of a licence or certificate and describes the process and possibility of appeal.
s. 14	forbids re-use of animals unless permission is given. (A)
s. 15	demands euthanasia at end of series of regulated procedures if suffering or likely adverse effects are present.
s. 16	prohibits use of protected animals in public displays.
s. 17	restricts the use of neuromuscular blocking agents.
s. 18	states the duties and powers of the Inspectors.
s. 19	describes the make-up of the Animal Procedures Committee (APC).
s. 20	states the function of the APC.
s. 21	presents miscellaneous and supplementary information on Guidance Notes, Codes of Practice, Information and Alterations by Parliamentary Resolutions, and the publishing of appropriate information.
s. 22	lists penalties under the Act.
s. 23	states penalties for making false statements.
s. 24	states penalties for disclosing confidential information.
s. 25	refers to entry of a constable with a warrant.
s. 26	refers to the process of prosecution under the Act.
s. 27	deals with repeal and consequential amendments in previous relevant Acts and transitional provisions in this Act, details of which appear in Sch. 3 and 4 of the Act.
s. 28	outlines the negative procedure associated with the enabling process of producing Statutory Instruments under this Act.
s. 29	deals with the application of the Act in N. Ireland.
s. 30	attends to routine legal matters, e.g. the title, interpretation and coming into force of the Act.

(A) These sections have been amended.

this case the relevant Secretary of State, the Home Secretary, is authorised to issue Statutory Instruments clarifying or amending but not of course radically changing the law as made and approved by Parliament.

Statutory Instruments

The definition of this term is complex and raises difficult points of interpretation. Broadly, the term covers delegated legislation made under:

(1) Powers conferred by statutes after 1947 on Her Majesty in Council, or on ministers or departments, to make, confirm or approve subordinate legislation where the enabling Act says that the power will be exercisable by Statutory Instrument.

(2) Powers conferred by statutes before 1948 on these authorities or other rule-making authorities (such as the Rule Committee of the Supreme Court) to make subordinate legislation, and on ministers to confirm or approve instruments of a legislative (but not of an executive) character which also have to be laid before Parliament.

(3) Regulations made by designated ministers under the European Communities Act 1972.

Government statements of policy and intent, departmental circulars giving instructions and procedural rules issued by certain other public bodies may be legislative in effect and will usually be published; but they will not be published as Statutory Instruments even if made in pursuance of statutory powers.

Under a few statutes, the initiative in preparing draft rules and regulations is given to bodies representing persons engaged in the occupation, and occasionally to individual so engaged; such schemes cannot normally be given legislative effect without the responsible minister's approval.

Statutory Instruments may appear in the form of Orders, Regulations and Rules.

The method of producing Statutory Instruments

The parent Act may or may not require the instruments to be laid before Parliament. If there is no requirement as to laying before Parliament, a member who gets to know about it may put down a question about it to the responsible minister. If the instrument is merely laid before Parliament, no opportunity is provided for it to be discussed, but at least it is brought to the notice of members. It is more common for the enabling Act to provide that an instrument shall be laid subject to the negative resolution procedure. It is then open to any member to move a prayer to annul the instrument.

A minority of instruments are required to be laid subject to an affirmative resolution of one or both Houses; unless a resolution approving the instrument is passed within the period (if any) prescribed by the enabling Act, the instrument ceases to have effect or, if only in draft, cannot be made.

Safeguards in respect to subordinate legislation

The most effective safeguard against the abuse of delegated legislation is caution with regard to the terms of delegation. The terms of delegation ought to be carefully worded. The established forms of prior consultation with advisory bodies and organised interest groups ought to be used to the full.

A Joint Select Committee was set up in 1977 to consider instruments laid before Parliament with a view to deciding whether the special attention of the House should be drawn to the instrument.

Knowing about Statutory Instruments

'Does any human being read through this mass of departmental legislation?' asked Lord Hewart (*The New Despotism* (1929), pp. 96–7). Unfortunately, *ignorantia juris neminem excusat* (ignorance of the law is no excuse). Statutory Instruments must be printed, numbered, published and sold. They are also published in annual volumes. However, local or temporary instruments, instruments made available in a separate series to persons directly concerned, and very bulky schedules may be exempted from the requirement of publication.

An instrument may nevertheless have legal effect before it is published and available for sale at a government bookshop but departments usually stipulate that an instrument shall not come into operation for 21 days after being laid before Parliament. It is, however, a defence to criminal proceedings for contravening an instrument to prove that the instrument had not been issued at the date of the contravention unless the prosecution proves that reasonable steps have previously been taken to bring its purport to the notice of the public or person likely to be affected (*Constitutional and Administrative Law*, S.A. de Smith, Penguin Books, 1978, pp. 328–35).

Delegated legislation and the 1986 Act

Fortunately, there has not been an abundance of delegated legislation associated with this Act, although one Statutory Instrument, in the form of an Order concerning appeal procedures, was issued even before the end of 1986. It was the Animals (Scientific Procedures) (Procedure for Representations) Rules 1986 (SI 1986/1911).

The delegation of legislative power to the Secretary of State occurs frequently throughout the Act:

(1) s. 1 (3) (a) and (b) – the protected animal;
(2) s. 2 (9) – euthanasia;
(3) s. 7 (9) – Sch. 2;
(4) s. 12 (7) – representation.

The following list (Table 2.2) illustrates the changing pattern of the legal control of the maintenance and use of animals in research during the 20 years since

Table 2.2   The enabling process and the changing pattern of practical aspects of A(SP)A

Year	Stage
1986	The first Statutory Instrument made under A(SP)A, The Animals (Scientific Procedures) (Procedure for Representations) Rules 1986 (SI 1986/1911). It was made on 7 November 1986 and laid before Parliament on 18 November, coming into operation on 10 December. This Statutory Instrument spelt out the details of the process for the relief of aggrieved parties under the A(SP)A. Production of *Guidance on the operation of A(SP)A*, a Code of Practice for the Housing and Care of Animals used in Scientific Procedures.
1987	Guidelines on eye irritation/corrosion tests. Guidelines on the use of neuromuscular blocking agents.
1989	Advice on research on psychological stress.
1990	Licensees past retirement age – restrictions.
1991	Antibody production – minimal severity. Advice guidelines on use of strychnine in research. Supplementary guidance notes on PPL for microsurgery training. Policy on laparoscopic surgery training.
1992	RCVS Code of Practice for NVSs.
1993	Quail (*Coturnix coturnix*) included in Sch. 2. Scientific procedures listing endangered species. Guidance on brokerage. Act extended to *Octopus vulgaris*.
1994	Code of Practice on licensing and inspection. Policy on conflict of interests of named persons. Revised guidelines on eye irritation tests. Training requirements for PIL applicants. Guidance on transgenics and harmful mutants.
1995	Training requirements for PPL applicants. Code of Practice for designated breeding and supplying establishments. New policy on the use of non-human primates. APC recommendations on regulatory toxicology testing. Revised system for reporting of annual statistics. Training requirements for NVSs.
1996	Requirements for the importation of primates to be used under the Act. Revision of Sch. 1 of the Act and the introduction of a Code of Practice on humane killing.
1997	Day-to-day care person renamed 'named animal care and welfare officer' (NACWO). Restrictions imposed on the use of the ascites method and cosmetic product, alcohol and tobacco testing.
1998	Comprehensive amendment of A(SP)A, particularly of ss. 4, 5, 10, 14 and the insertion of Sch. 2a. These changes are given in detail in the Schedule to the Statutory Instrument, Animals (Scientific Procedures) Act 1986 (Amendment) Regulations 1998 which came into force in

Cont.

Table 2.2 Cont.

Year	Stage
	1998. The main effects of this amendment appear to be a requirement for proven competency on the part of PIL holders (s. 4), necessity always to consider seriously the 3 Rs (s. 5), provision for keeping animals after procedure, possibility of release, stipulations on the marking of animals and control of the use of animals from the wild (s. 10), greater restriction on the re-use of animals (s. 14) and emphasis on the need to use anaesthetics (Sch. 2a). These amendments were introduced to bring our law into greater conformity with the Council Directive 86/609/EEC (OJ No L358 18 December 1986 p. 1). This text will reflect the amendment as the occasion arises. In 1998 there were further restrictions of testing of ingredients of cosmetics. Upgrading of dog facilities was also introduced. LERP (cf. PCD 4/98).
1999	Ferret, gerbil, genetically modified pig and genetically modified sheep became Sch. 2 animals. (1 Jan. 1999). Call for listing in designated establishments of those competent in the operation of Sch. 1 methods. Compulsory local ethical review process as from 1 April 1999.
2000	Introduction of new Home Office Guidance. Implementation of new Licensing Charter. Implementation of three-tier system for handling infringements. European Commission approve three alternative tests as scientifically validated, for skin corrosivity testing – TER and EPISKIN and 3T3 NRA relating to phototoxic potential. Re-derivation of conventional animals to manage stock or eradicate welfare problems is to be regarded as husbandry/veterinary practice. Imported embryos to be coded in the annual return according to their place of birth, i.e. as UK animals. Cross–Whitehall concordat on data sharing. Revised form of Project Licence Application Form with full Guidance Notes introduced. Guidance on Regulatory Toxicity Testing issued. Exemption from some Home Office Training requirements for holders of evidence of FELASA training.
2001	Production of a Supplementary Guidance on the production of antibodies as a service. European Commission recommends a Good Practice Guide to the Administration of Substances and Removal of Blood produced by European Federation of Pharmaceutical Industries Associations (EFPIA) and the European Centre for the Validation of Alternative Methods (ECVAM). Booklet published by LAVA on the Discharge of Animals from the A(SP)A recommended by the Home Office. New application form for authority to transfer animals. Guidance on the Conduct of Regulatory Toxicology and Safety Evaluation Studies appears on Home Office website. Publication of a further and broader Guide on Administration of Substances, *Laboratory Animals* (2001) 35: 1–41.

Cont.

Table 2.2   Cont.

Year	Stage
2002	Code of Practice Supplement for Ferrets and Gerbils.
	Council of Europe approve a Protocol Amendment to European Convention ETS 123 to enable a simple procedure to amend the Convention's technical Appendices, for example the Appendix on standards of animal accommodation and care.
	Publication of the House of Lords Select Committee on Animals in Scientific Procedures with recommendations to develop application of the 3Rs, to streamline licensing process and to provide more information for the public.
	Organisation for Economic Co-operation and Development (OECD) adopted the murine Local Lymph Node Assay in place of the guinea pig maximisation test for skin sensitisation which would now demand specific scientific justification.
	Health and Safety Inspection of Animal Facilities to reduce risk of Laboratory Animal Allergies (LAA).
	HO Guidance Note on Non-Rodent Selection in Pharmaceutical Toxicology.
2003	Rejection of the House of Lords Select Committee's recommendation that each ERP should contain an external lay member. The HO, however, do urge Certificate Holders to increase lay representation on their ERP.
	The Inter-Departmental Data Sharing Group become the Inter-Departmental Group on the 3Rs.
	The Technical Expert Working Group (TWEG) commence revision of Directive 86/609/EC. The Chief Inspector represented the HO.
	Revision of the Code of Practice for Named Veterinary Surgeons.
	HO supports the work of the Medical Research Centre for Best Practice for Animals in Research (CBPAR).
	Revision of the import conditions and application form for the import of rodent embryos, ova and semen (cf. DEFRA).
	HO Guidance Note on Water and Food Restriction for Scientific Purposes.
2004	Introduction of mandatory training for NACWOs.
	Publication of Tewg's report on revision of Directive 86/609/EEC.
	APC recommends extending protection of A(SP)A to all octopus, squid and cuttlefish. It also recommends amendment of Sch.1.
	Publication of Abstracts of project licence applications.
2005	HO draws attention to Guidelines on the Care and Use of Fish in Research issued by the Canadian Council on Animal Care (CCAC) and to the work of the National Centre for the Replacement, Refinement and Reduction of Animals in Research (NC3Rs).
	New Project Licence Application Form with electronic format and detailed Guidance Notes.
2006	Parties to the Council of Europe Convention ETS 123 adopt revised text of Appendix A. Provisions to take effect from 15 June 2007.
	Direction that ERP documents should be attached to the Certificate of Designation.

the enactment of the A(SP)A. Most of the topics referred to will be commented upon in the text where appropriate.

I have been able to compile this collection of the results of the enabling process and of relevant and even peripheral stipulations concerning animals in research due to a generous supply from the HO of PCDs. PCDs are helpful pieces of information issued by the HO to Certificate Holders several times a year.

Not just the Home Office

The administration of Statutory Instruments and other legislation regarding animals is not solely confined to the Home Office. Other organs of government are involved in controlling animal use and welfare, and in dealing with legal matters that are relevant to the proper running of animal units. Some of these affairs will be dealt with by the devolved administrations of Scotland, Wales and Northern Ireland.

Some of the branches of government which should be considered as relevant, with examples of their area of concern, are shown in Table 2.3.

Table 2.3   Some of the branches of government and their areas of concern relating to animals

Department	Example
Department of the Environment, Food and Rural Affairs (DEFRA)	Animal Health and Wildlife
Department of Health (DH)	Medicines Act 1968
Department of Health in Northern Ireland	Animals (Scientific Procedures) Act 1986
Local government authorities	Collection and Disposal of Waste Regulations 1988
Local constabulary	Firemans Act 1968
Commissioners of Revenues & Customs	Endangered Species (Import and Export)

If no specific arm of government is directly concerned with a piece of legislation then the usual legal processes come into operation in the prosecution of an offence, for example prosecution by the Crown Prosecution Service or a private prosecution or, in civil cases, a suing of the defendant by a claimant (for instance, under the Animals Act 1971).

Chapter 3

The Protected Animal

'Protected animal' defined

The crucial definition of 'protected animal' in s. 1 of the A(SP)A was amended by a Statutory Instrument, in keeping with the enabling powers of the Secretary of State as stated:

's. 1(1) Subject to the provisions of this section . . .'

and

's. 1(3) The Secretary of State may by order:

(a) extend the definition of protected animal so as to include invertebrates of any description;'

The Animals (Scientific Procedures) Act (Amendment) Order 1993 extended the original definition of 'protected animal' (only vertebrates) to an invertebrate species. The definition of 'protected animal' now reads:

'A "protected animal" for the purposes of this Act means any living vertebrate and any invertebrate of the species *Octopus vulgaris* from the stage of its development when it becomes capable of independent feeding.'

A comprehensive treatment of the arguments leading to the insertion of the *Octopus vulgaris* into this definition appeared in the 1992 APC Report, pp. 7–8.

For the purposes of the Act, an animal is regarded as 'living' until the permanent cessation of circulation or the destruction of the brain. Brain destruction is not complete in decerebrated animals; these are considered to be living and are protected under the Act.

For clarification of 'destruction of the brain', refer to the Code of Practice dealt with later in association with Schedule 1.

An animal becomes protected when it reaches the following stages of development:

- in the case of mammals, birds and reptiles halfway through gestation or incubation periods;

- in the case of fish, amphibians and *Octopus vulgaris* the time at which they become capable of independent feeding.

The Secretary of State is enabled by s. 1(3)(b) to alter the stage of development at which an animal may become protected.

There are animals and animals

In the amended (1998) s. 5(5)(b) of A(SP)A a sort of grading of animals was introduced:

'that the regulated procedures to be used are those which . . . involve animals with the lowest degree of neurophysiological sensitivity, . . .'

Special justification is looked for in the case of the use of cats, dogs, equidae and primates. In the amended s. 10(6) of A(SP)A attention is drawn to the need for special identification of dogs, cats and primates.

Increasingly, and rightly so, emphasis has been laid on the need to avoid the use of primates in research whenever possible.

The *LASA Newsletter* (Winter 1997) refers to the limitations on the use of primates:

'Great apes have never been used under the 1986 Act as laboratory animals. In future the Government will not allow their use. It is felt that the cognitive and behavioural characteristics of these animals means it is unethical to treat them as expendable for research.

It was also confirmed that wild-caught primates of any species will only be allowed in scientific procedures if exceptionally justified. For wild-caught primates to be authorized, there must be no alternative tests appropriate, no suitable captive-bred animals available and the likely benefit must fully justify their use.'

Chapter 4

The Regulated Procedure

Section 2(1) of the A(SP)A states:

> 'Subject to the provisions of this section, "a regulated procedure" for the purposes of this Act means any experimental or other scientific procedure applied to a protected animal which may have the effect of causing that animal pain, suffering, distress or lasting harm.'

The Home Office Guidance on the Operation of the Animals (Scientific Procedures) Act expounds on the connotation and extension of the term, 'regulated procedure'. (Guidance 2.13–23)

The terms 'pain, suffering, distress or lasting harm' include death, disease, injury, physiological and psychological stress, significant discomfort, or any disturbance to normal health, whether immediately or in the long term.

A procedure may be regulated if composed of a combination of non-regulated techniques which may cause pain, suffering, distress or lasting harm. The legal distinction between a procedure and a technique is not clarified.

A procedure is regulated if, following or during a procedure, an animal reaches the stage at which it becomes a protected animal and the procedure may have the effect of causing pain, suffering, distress or lasting harm.

A procedure which may result in pain, suffering, distress or lasting harm to a foetus or immature form at or beyond the stage at which it becomes protected is regarded as a regulated procedure, irrespective of any effect on the parent animal. Anything which may result in the birth or hatching of a protected animal with abnormalities which may cause it pain, suffering, distress or lasting harm (for instance, the breeding of animals with harmful genetic defects) is a regulated procedure. It follows that the term 'regulated procedure' can include genetic manipulation involving animals which will reach the stage at which they will become protected animals. The crucial term 'may' in the definition of regulated procedure is of importance in this context.

A procedure is still regulated even if any pain, suffering, distress or lasting harm which would have otherwise resulted is mitigated or prevented by anaesthetics or other substances to sedate, restrain, or dull perception, or by prior decerebration or other procedure for rendering the animal insentient.

The giving of an anaesthetic or analgesic or other substance to sedate or dull the perception of pain of a protected animal for scientific purposes is itself a regulated procedure. Likewise, decerebration, or any other procedure to render a protected animal insentient, if done for scientific purposes, is a regulated procedure.

The comments on the definition of a regulated procedure in the Guidance are useful and significant because a clear grasp of this term is crucial to the proper understanding of the A(SP)A. If one is involved in a regulated procedure one needs authorisation in the form of licences and the appropriate certificate. If what is being done to the animal is not a 'regulated procedure', no licence is required.

The purpose of the procedure, as well as the level of suffering caused, determines whether or not licence authorities under the Act are required. For example, the taking of a blood sample or the forceful removal of a feather to provide material solely to identify an individual, or its provenance, would not be regulated under the Act. However, the same type of sampling to provide data for an experimental or other scientific purpose (for example, to study population dynamics or to determine whether or not the animal had been genetically modified) would be regulated by the Act.

The Home Office should be consulted when there is any doubt as to whether a proposed intervention is regulated by the Act. (Guidance 2.34–35)

A clarification of the interpretation of the law as regards water and food restriction for scientific purposes was issued as a special Guidance Note on 20 November 2003.

Where possible traditional food and water restriction paradigms should be replaced by reward paradigms and only if this is found, or is known, to be inappropriate should restriction paradigms be considered.

As a general rule when undertaken for a scientific purpose, all food restriction should be kept to the absolute minimum required to achieve the scientific objective. Project Licence authority which clearly justifies the work and the benefits that should result will be required for:

- all work which restricts food intake to a point where weight loss, or reduced weight gain, of more that 15% of age and sex matched non-deprived animals might occur; or
- all work where animals are to be maintained below 85% of body weight for age and sex matched controls fed ad libitum.

This guidance does not apply to simple dietary studies in farm animals, which will be covered separately.

Water should be made available ad libitum at all times. Water withholding is not regulated when it is removed as part of recognised husbandry practices. Regulation under the Animals (Scientific Procedures) Act 1986 (A(SP)A) is necessary when the programme of work to be applied requires water withdrawal that may result in pain, suffering, distress and lasting harm and is applied for a scientific purpose.

For guidance

With respect to food restriction, current Home Office guidance, as applied to Schedule 2 listed species, and ruminants, recommends that as long as no additional factor other than food deprivation is applied, exceeding the following food deprivation times for scientific purposes requires Project Licence authority:

16 hours – mice, young hamsters and rats under 100gms

24 hours – rabbits, rats, dogs, cats and non-human primates weighing over 100gms

See Note 1: Adult ruminants and other farm animals (including chickens and turkeys).

Note 1: The Home Office considers that any restriction of food and water for a scientific purpose which would breach other welfare legislation (e.g. Welfare of Farmed Animals England [SI 1870] or Northern Ireland [SI 270] Regulations) or current DEFRA Welfare Codes for that species will require regulation under A(SP)A.

Note 2: Food restriction should be avoided in guinea pigs, ferrets and shrews.

Note 3: The deprivation of food or water combined with one or more additional factor(s) (e.g. high-protein diet, concurrent disease) may require a reduction in these times if additional suffering is considered likely.

Note 4: Authority is also required if animals are exposed to repeated daily periods of deprivation shorter than detailed in the table above.

Scientists using water restriction should keep the following records for each animal:

- daily water consumption, food consumption, body weight
- frequency of surgical intervention (if appropriate)
- frequency of infections/treatments (if appropriate)
- duration of study and future plans for the animal (if appropriate)
- a record of all treatments given.

Unless there is a veterinary contraindication or a justified scientific reason for not doing so, animals should be returned to ad libitum water at least 24 hours before a procedure that requires anaesthesia and should remain on ad libitum water for at least 48 hours after the conclusion of the procedure. Water provision must also be increased when an animal:

- is showing clinical signs of dehydration
- is treated for disease
- is exhibiting a weight loss
- is young and is failing to gain a reasonable weight increase during the time when it should be growing
- is considered, by a veterinary surgeon, to be compromised because of some other circumstance.

Variation in the acceptability of some procedures

A government policy announcement appeared in the 1997 Report (p. 5, n. 37) of the APC.

'37. In November, the Government issued a supplementary note to its response on our interim report in which it published a policy statement on the use of animals in scientific procedures. It promised:

- an end to the use of animals in the testing of finished cosmetic products had been secured through a voluntary agreement with the companies carrying out this type of work in the UK.
- the possibility of ending the use of animals in testing finished household products and the testing of ingredients for the types of cosmetics which could be called 'vanity products' would be explored; [In 1998 a ban was imposed on the testing of the ingredients of cosmetics on animals.]
- tests which involved animals in the testing of offensive weapons, or of alcohol or tobacco products would not be allowed;
- the use of ascetic animals in the production of monoclonal anti-bodies would be phased out.'

Procedures which are not regulated

The words of the Act 'subject to the provisions of this section' (A(SP)A s. 2(1)) allow for exceptions in law as regards some scientific procedures on animals.

In keeping with subsections (5), (6), (7) and (8) of s. 1 there are procedures which appear to have the three essential elements of a regulated procedure – 'scientific', 'a protected animal' and 'pain'. They are not, however, regulated procedures because the law says they are not. Description of these exempt procedures is given in Guidance 2.24–2.34.

(1) Ringing, tagging or marking of an animal or any other humane procedure for the sole purpose of enabling an animal to be identified, if it causes only momentary pain or distress or no lasting harm.
(2) Clinical testing on animals for evaluation of a veterinary product in accordance with the Medicines Act 1968.
(3) Procedures carried out for the purposes of recognised veterinary, agricultural or animal husbandry practice are not regulated under the Act. For example, taking blood or other tissue samples for diagnosis and giving established medicines by injection are recognised veterinary procedures, if done for the benefit of the animal. Similarly, husbandry practices which may cause pain, such as castration, are not regulated procedures unless they form part of a scientific study. Where there is doubt, the Inspector should be consulted. This is wise advice. From experience it is apparent that official interpretation may vary in this matter.
(4) Euthanasia by a Schedule 1 method is not a regulated procedure.

Chapter 5

Schedule 1 of the A(SP)A

Schedules are usually lists of relevant legislative detail appended to an Act. Although placed at the end of an Act, they have equal legal force with any section of the Act. Indeed the sole prosecution under the Act for more than the first ten years of the A(SP)A was for a breach of Schedule 2. This case will be referred to later in association with Schedule 2. The current Schedules to the A(SP)A are shown in Table 5.1.

Table 5.1 The five schedules of the A(SP)A

Sch. 1	(Revised 1996) Appropriate methods of humane killing.
Sch. 2	(Revised 1993 and 1998) List of animals to be obtained only from designated breeding or supplying establishments. This Schedule will be commented upon in the chapter on certificates of designation.
Sch. 3	Consequential amendments. The aim of this Schedule was the replacement of references in earlier Acts to the Cruelty to Animals Act 1876 by references to the Animals (Scientific Procedures) Act 1986.
Sch. 4	Transitional provisions dealing with delays in bringing into operation certain parts of the Act. These adjustments are, of course, all now completed. Most of them, e.g. the implementation of Sch. 2 and replacements of 1876 licences, were in place before 1990.
Sch. 2a	A requirement to use anaesthetics in all experiments on animals unless there are irrefutable reasons for acting otherwise. This new Sch. 2a, which is not associated with Sch. 2, was issued with the amended form of A(SP)A published towards the end of 1998. This Schedule will be expounded upon along with the amended and augmented conditions on the personal licence.

The force of Schedule 1

The implication of Schedule 1 is that if an animal in a designated establishment is killed by a method approved for that type of animal, that killing is not a regulated procedure and so no licence is needed to cause legally the death of that animal.

The person performing this procedure, however, must be competent in that method of euthanasia. Any uncertainty consequent on the lack of a clear definition of 'competent' has now been obviated by the demand for the drawing up of a register in designated establishments of persons competent in the approved methods of killing in the particular establishment. There is a comment on this aspect of Schedule 1 in the 1997 Report (p. 109, nn. 13–14) of the APC.

'13. We also note that, for those who believe that their particular circumstances merit the use of a humane method not described in Schedule 1, the necessary authority can be granted in the relevant certificate.'

(If this is in the context of a dedicated breeding or supplying establishment it would seem there could be the possibility of a personal licensee operating outside the scope of a project licence, unless it was a case of killing animals of a mutant strain expressing a defective gene or genetically manipulated animals.)

'14. There were also concerns about the qualifications and competence of those undertaking Schedule 1 killing. The Home Office has already accepted the recommendations that we made in our interim report that those carrying out Schedule 1 killings should be appropriately trained and that establishments be required to maintain a register of those competent to humanely kill animals.'

Schedule 1 in detail

Appropriate methods of humane killing

(A(SP)A s. 2, 6, 7, 10, 15(1) and 18(3))

'1. Subject to paragraph 2 below, the methods of humane killing listed in Tables A and B below are appropriate for the animals listed in the corresponding entries in those tables only if the process of killing is completed by one of the methods listed in sub-paragraphs (a) to (f) below:
(a)   confirmation of permanent cessation of the circulation
(b)   destruction of the brain
(c)   dislocation of the neck
(d)   exsanguination
(e)   confirming the onset of rigor mortis
(f)   instantaneous destruction of the body in a macerator.

2. Paragraph 1 above does not apply in those cases where Table A specifies one of the methods listed in that paragraph as an appropriate method of humane killing.

A. **Methods for animals other than foetal, larval and embryonic forms**	**Animals for which appropriate**
1. Overdose of an anaesthetic using a route and an anaesthetic agent appropriate for the size and species of animal	All animals
2. Exposure to carbon dioxide gas in a rising concentration	Rodents, rabbits and birds up to 1.5 kg
3. Dislocation of the neck	Rodents up to 500 g Rabbits up to 1 kg Birds up to 3 kg
4. Concussion of the brain by striking the cranium	Rodents and rabbits up to 1 kg Birds up to 250 g Amphibians and reptiles up to 1 kg (with destruction of the brain before the return of consciousness) Fishes (with destruction of the brain before the return of consciousness)
5. One of the recognised methods of slaughter set out below which is appropriate to the animal and is performed by a registered veterinary surgeon, or, in the case of the methods described in paragraph (ii) below, performed by the holder of a current licence granted under the Welfare of Animals (Slaughter or Killing) Regulations 1995 (a). (i) Destruction of the brain by free bullet, or (ii) captive bolt, percussion or electrical stunning followed by destruction of the brain or exsanguinations before the return of consciousness.	Ungulates

B. Methods for foetal, larval and embryonic forms	**Animals for which appropriate**
1. Overdose of an anaesthetic using a route and anaesthetic agent appropriate for the size, stage of development and species of animal.	All animals
2. Refrigeration, or disruption of membranes, or maceration in apparatus approved under appropriate slaughter legislation, or exposure to carbon dioxide in near 100% concentration until they are dead	Birds Reptiles
3. Cooling of foetuses followed by immersion in cold tissue fixative	Mice, rats and rabbits
4. Decapitation	Mammals and birds up to 50 g

(a) S.I. 1995/731'

Code of practice for the humane killing of animals under Schedule 1 to the Animals (Scientific Procedures) Act 1986

One marked advantage of this new form of Schedule 1 has been the addition of a code of practice providing commentary on and explanation of the terms used in the Schedule.

For a full grasp of what is involved, the actual text of both the Code and the Schedule should be studied. The material in Table 5.2 is merely intended to high-light more significant material from parts of the Code.

There is the possibility that Schedule 1 might be amended again, particularly the attached code of practice. This would be due to the growing emphasis on the concept of 'Good Practice' and the need to employ it in every aspect of the use and maintenance of animals in research.

Laboratory animal science abounds with material questioning some of the approved methods of killing animals, especially the use of a long-standing method, that is, the use of carbon dioxide. A Statutory Instrument (2000 No. 3352) issued by MAFF, of happy memory, had already commenced to alter methods of euthanasia in farming in consideration of new attitudes to established methods. Refer to The Amendment of the Welfare of Animals (Slaughter or Killing) Regulations 1995. (For this and future similar SIs, refer to www.opsi.gov.uk/stat.htm.)

Table 5.2   Code of Practice under Schedule 1 to A(SP)A

Part 1 is a general introduction

Part 2 refers to the various stipulations in the Act on euthanasia; most of this material occurs elsewhere in this work but some items call for special attention:

- 'Killing a protected animal for a scientific purpose at a designated establishment does not require a licence if a method listed in Schedule 1, appropriate to the animal, is used. However, if another method is used the killing is a regulated procedure and requires personal and project licence authority.' (2.1) This statement is crucial to the proper understanding of the legal implications of this Schedule 1.
- 'Under Section 10(2)(b) of the Act there is an inviolable termination condition applied as condition 14 to all personal licences. If an animal undergoing a regulated procedure shows signs of severe pain or distress which cannot be alleviated, the personal licensee must ensure that it is killed painlessly without delay . . .' (2.7)
- The executive power of the Inspector to require the killing of an animal if he/she considers it is undergoing excessive suffering carries a criminal sanction. (2.8)

Part 3 is concerned with safeguards for humane killing, e.g.:

- Sympathetic handling is paramount. (3.1)
- Do not kill animal in the presence of others. (3.2)
- Adjust the method to cause the least amount of suffering, induce terminal unconsciousness. (3.3)
- Only those who are competent should use physical methods of killing animals. (3.4)
- The CH should ensure the competency of those members of staff who are required to kill animals. (3.5)
- 'It is accepted that killing a pregnant animal by a Schedule 1 method in the later stages of gestation normally leads to the death of the fetus. There is no evidence to suggest that the death of the unborn animal would be distressful and inhumane provided direct physical injury to the fetus is avoided. Killing the pregnant dam by a Schedule 1 method does not require licence authority. Project and personal licence authority is required to use the live fetus in a regulated procedure after the half-way stage of gestation.' (3.7)

Part 4 demands confirmation of death before disposal and describes ways of ensuring the animal is dead, e.g.:

- Check circulation has ceased from the absence of pulse or heart beat or make certain of death by section of the heart or great vessels. (4.2, 4.5)
- The permanent loss of function rather than physical destruction of brain structure can be confirmed by no reflex to stimulus, e.g. by touching the cornea, or by the cessation of breathing. (4.3)
- Death from dislocation of the neck can be confirmed by palpation. (4.4)
- Observation of rigor mortis can be used to ensure that death has occurred. (4.6)
- When macerators are used for the disposal of small carcasses, there must be confirmation that there is no longer any response to any painful stimulus. (4.7)

Part 5 refers to various obligations in respect of the disposal of carcasses such as:

- To be sure the animal is dead. (5.1)
- To dispose on site if possible or discreetly. (5.2)
- To comply with all statutory legislation on the disposal of hazardous material. (5.3)
- To comply with special conditions in disposing of the carcasses of farm animals. (5.4)

Cont.

Table 5.2 Cont.

Part 6 comments on the appropriate methods of humane killing in practice:

- Training or in some cases special qualifications (e.g. licensed slaughtermen or veterinary surgeons) are required. (6.1)
- The guidance given in Part 6 is neither comprehensive nor mandatory. (6.2)
- When an anaesthetic is used the method, route and agent must be the most appropriate to the particular animal and there should be rapid loss of consciousness. (A.1)
- Direct injection into the heart can be painful and should not be used. (A.1)
- Anaesthesia induced by inhalation is not suitable for large animals nor diving animals. In the case of small animals care must be taken in administering anaesthetic inhalants and an effective scavenging system must be in place. (A.1)
- The recommended method of euthanasia for fish, amphibia and *Octopus vulgaris* is immersion in water containing an appropriate anaesthetic agent. (A.1)
- Details are given for the proper use of carbon dioxide gas for euthanasia e.g. the chamber should be emptied and flushed clear after each batch of animals has been killed. (A.2)
- Special training and skill is required for killing by dislocation of the neck. (A.3)
- Killing by concussion calls for special expertise and a great amount of care and attention is needed to ensure immediate death. (A.4)
- The use of a free bullet, captive bolt, percussion or electric stunning requires specialised equipment and approved expert operators. (A.5)
- Some small fetuses, embryos and larvae can be killed by immersion in anaesthetic agents. (B.1)
- Euthanasia by refrigeration of chick embryos can be by exposure to 4°C or below for more than four hours. (B.2)
- Chick embryos can be killed by passing the eggs through a macerator similar to those used for day old chicks and unhatched eggs – see EC Regulation COM(91)136. Intact embryonated eggs and exposed embryos or larvae can be killed by keeping them in near 100% carbon dioxide gas for a long time until they are dead.'(B.2)
- In the case of reptilian embryos death should be ensured by an overdose of an anaesthetic agent, maceration or immersion in a tissue fixative. (B.2)
- Tissues fixative used in the euthanasia of fetuses should be 4°C. (B.3)
- Decapitation can be carried out with a strong pair of sharp scissors. (B.4)

Chapter 6

The Personal Licence

Definition of the personal licence

'A personal licence is the Secretary of State's endorsement that the holder is
a suitable and competent person to carry out, under supervision if necessary,
specified procedures on specified classes of animal (Section 3).

It does not authorize the holder to carry out any regulated procedure unless
this is part of the programme of work authorized by a project licence
(Section 3). The place of work must be stipulated in both the personal and
project licence.'

(Guidance 6.1–2)

Except when issued to students and others for the purposes of study, personal licences,
unless they are revoked, generally remain in force indefinitely.

They must be reviewed at intervals of not more than five years (s. 4(5)). Other
than when the review is brought forward to coincide with an amendment request,
the personal licensee will be advised when the review process is being undertaken
and requested to confirm the appropriateness of personal details, authorised techniques and species, and additional conditions. The APC recommended in its 1990
Report (nn. 28–33) restrictions, limiting the licences of those approaching 70 years
of age.

The crucial consideration taken into account in the issuing of a personal licence
is competence. It is an appropriate skill or technique which is required. On the
other hand, in the case of a project licence, the establishment of justification
is demanded in the application and the ability to fulfil a managerial role is all-
important.

Qualifications

'An applicant for a personal licence must:
- be at least 18 years of age [Section 4(4)]
- have appropriate education and training (including instruction in a relevant scientific discipline) and experience for the purpose of competently
  handling the protected animals, applying the specified regulated procedures

to the specified classes of animal, and taking responsibility thereafter for the welfare of the animals [Section 4(4A)]: and

- be competent to apply those techniques in accordance with the conditions included in the licence [Section 4(4A)].

A personal licence applicant will normally be expected to provide evidence of appropriate education, training and experience. Typically this will comprise:

- at least five GCSEs or Standard Grade passes (including a biological science), or equivalent vocational qualifications; and
- a certificate attesting to successful completion of training modules 1, 2 and 3 for the relevant species; and, in appropriate cases, module 4.'

(Guidance Appendix F)

'Applicants may request exemption from these requirements if suitable evidence is supplied of comparable education, training or experience.'

(Guidance 6.3–5)

Note: the sections referred to are those of the Animals (Scientific Procedures) Act.

Sponsorship

'A personal licence applicant must normally be sponsored by a personal licence holder who holds a position of authority at the place where the applicant is to be authorized by the licence to carry out regulated procedures [Section 4(3)]. The sponsor must be able to certify that the applicant's qualifications and character are satisfactory for the work for which a licence is sought, and that the appropriate accredited training has been successfully undertaken or that any exemptions requested from the general training requirements are justified and supported.

When an applicant does not have English as a first language, the sponsor is expected to confirm that the applicant understands the provisions of the Act.'

(Guidance 6.6–7)

Supervision

'Until technical proficiency and competence are attained, the Secretary of State requires that the personal licensee accepts supervision and training arrangements put in place by the project licence holder, or by competent personal licensees nominated by the project licence holder. The limits of supervisory responsibility should be clear to all involved. The level and extent of necessary supervision and training should be reviewed and agreed periodically by the project and personal licence holders.'

'The Home Office regards this as an important responsibility of project licence holders and expects them to be able to demonstrate that appropriate supervision and training are actively provided for the licensees working under their direction and control.'

'Generally, personal licensees are not restricted to work under the project licence specified at the time the application is made. They may, unless restricted by a condition of issue on the personal licence, work under any project licence at the designated establishments at which their personal licence is valid providing the techniques and species to be used are authorized on their personal licence and they are working under the direction and control of the relevant project licence holder.'

(Guidance 6.9)

Responsibilities of the personal licence holder

The responsibilities of the personal licence holder can be ascertained from the 22 conditions attached to the licence. The Inspectorate can, of course, attach additional appropriate conditions to any licence or certificate if circumstances demand it. The full text of licence and certificate conditions is at the back of this book.

There are, however, important responsibilities associated with the personal licence which merit special attention.

According to COPHCASP (Code of Practice for The Housing and Care of Animals used in Scientific Procedures) (para. 3.4) the personal licence holder bears primary responsibility for the care of all animals submitted to procedures under the terms of his or her licence. This demands the personal licence holder's presence at any time when an animal is most likely to be in pain or distress, especially when recovering from a procedure or under an anaesthetic.

The Guidance (6.18) clarifies the situation where more than one personal licensee may be involved with the same animal.

'Where two or more personal licensees have applied regulated procedures to the same animal (for example, one person surgically prepares the animal and another licensee later administers test substances), it must be clear at all times which licensee has primary responsibility for the animal. Normally, responsibility is retained by the licensee who applied the last of the regulated procedures.'

It is the responsibility of the personal licensee to familiarise themselves with the severity limit of procedures listed in the project licence in the protocol sheet 19a and the constraints upon adverse effects described in the protocol sheet 19b.

Personal licensees should ensure that the cages, pens or places in which the animals are held carry labels indicating the project licence number, the responsible personal licensee's number, the procedures which the animals are undergoing, when the procedures commenced and any additional information which may be required by the Inspector.

Large animals, as well as cats and dogs and all non-human primates, must be individually identified.

An understanding of the subordinate position of some personal licensees within some structures is shown in the A(SP)A (s. 22(4)).

'A person shall not be guilty of an offence under section 3 or 17(a) above' (these sections stipulate the need for the authority of a project licence to perform a regulated procedure and for the authority of a project licence to use a neuromuscular blocking agent) 'by reason, only that he acted without the authority of a project licence if he shows that he reasonably believed, after making due enquiry, that he had such authority.'

This is not a complete reneging on the solid legal principle – *ignorantia juris neminem excusat* (ignorance of the law excuses no man) – but is rather a very sensible provision for cases of ignorance of fact where juniors might be unduly influenced and misled by forcefully expressed opinions of their seniors.

Guidelines on neuromuscular blocking agents

The following extract from the APC Report 1988, pp. 26–28, sums up the legal position. For further details consult the Guidance Appendix K.

'3. In section 17 of the Animals (Scientific Procedures) Act 1986 it states that "no person shall in the course of a regulated procedure:
(a) use any neuromuscular blocking agent unless expressly authorized to do so by the personal and project licences under which the procedure is carried out; or
(b) use any such agent as an anaesthetic."
To do so would constitute an offence under the Act. But should a person be able to show that he reasonably believed after making due enquiry that he had appropriate authority, he would not be guilty of the offence in (a) above.

4. Neuromuscular blocking agents may be classified according to their action at the motor endplate:
(a) depolarising – including suxamethonium.
(b) non-polarising – including tubocurarine, gallamine, alcuronium, pancuronium, atracurium, and vecuronium.'

5. There are other naturally occurring biological compounds, such as venoms (e.g. Black Widow Spider) and toxins (e.g. *Clostridium botulinum* toxin) which when used systematically block neuromuscular transmission. There are also other agents (e.g. neomycin, high concentrations of magnesium ions) which have non-specific effects at the motor endplate. Such agents are not used clinically as neuromuscular blockers, and neither is it intended that they should be used instead of an anaesthetic. They will not be regarded specifically as neuromuscular blocking agents for the purpose of the Animals (Scientific Procedures) Act 1986; however, they must not be administered to living animals

for an experimental or other scientific purpose unless authorized by a project licence.'

Applicants intending to use muscular blocking agents will need to understand their use as set out in the relevant guidelines. They will normally be required to have witnessed their use and be familiar with the procedures for achieving and maintaining anaesthesia under such regimes. Where a licensee has been given permission to use neuromuscular blocking agents for the first time, he/she will, unless specifically exempted by the Home Secretary, be required to give the Inspector 48 hours' notice of the procedure. This restriction may be extended to further occasions if the Inspector considers it appropriate.

'8. These personal and project licence requirements do not apply to the use of such blocking agents during licensed work performed on decerebrate animals.'

Schedule 2A

Schedule 2A resulted from the October 1998 amendment of A(SP)A (s. 10(2a)). This amendment was an implementation of Article 8 of Council Directive No. 86/609/EEC.

'1.   All experiments shall be carried out under general or local anaesthesia.
2.   Paragraph 1 above does not apply when:
     (a)   anaesthesia is judged to be more traumatic to the animal than the experiment itself;
     (b)   anaesthesia is incompatible with the object of the experiment. In such cases appropriate legislative and/or administrative measures shall be taken to ensure that no such experiment is carried out unnecessarily.
     Anaesthesia should be used in the case of serious injuries which may cause severe pain.
3.   If anaesthesia is not possible, analgesics or other appropriate methods should be used in order to ensure as far as possible that pain, suffering, distress or harm are limited and that in any event the animal is not subject to severe pain, distress or suffering.
4.   Provided such action is compatible with the object of the experiment, an anaesthetised animal, which suffers considerable pain once anaesthesia has worn off, shall be treated in good time with pain–relieving means or, if this is not possible, shall be immediately killed by a humane method.'

Condition 19A on the personal licence enforces paras 1 and 2 of Schedule 2A but 'authorized procedure' (with a wider connotation) replaces 'experiment'. Condition 19B enforces para. 4 of Schedule 2A. Condition 19C enforces para. 3 of Schedule 2A.

Non-technical Procedures

'If the conditions of a personal licence permit the holder to use assistants to perform, under his direction, tasks not requiring technical knowledge nothing done by an assistant in accordance with such condition shall constitute a contravention of Section 3.'

(cf. A(SP)A s. 10(4)).

Permission to use assistants is sought by ticking the 'yes' box in section 16 of the application form for a personal licence. The specific authority to delegate, granted in response to this request, will be contained in the personal licence. The terms of such a condition on the personal licence must be strictly observed.

Guidance 6.22–27 provides a list, but not an exhaustive list, of 'some examples' of the kind of tasks which may be delegated. There is no attempt to define these 'non-technical procedures'; rather it is a matter of giving 'for instances' – perhaps rightly so, because rigid definitions fossilise law and obviate desirable flexibility in its application. The Inspector will readily advise on these matters. Some examples of permitted assistance in transgenic work might not be regarded by some as non-technical in ordinary parlance.

Where the list below of the non-technical procedures refers to tasks 'previously' carried out, those tasks will have been specified by a suitably qualified personal licensee, who must be within reach for assistance or advice if required.

'1)	The filling of food hoppers and water bottles with previously mixed diets or liquids of altered constitution or to which test substances have been previously added.

2)	The placing of animals in some previously set-up altered environments, e.g. inhalation chambers, pressure chambers, aquatic environments.

3)	Pressing the exposure button to deliver previously determined doses of irradiation to an animal.

4)	Pairing/grouping associated with the breeding of animals with harmful genetic defects.

5)	Withdrawal of contents from an established ruminal fistula.

6)	Operating automated machinery which carries out inoculation of eggs.

7)	Placement of animals in restraining devices, as defined by the project licence.

8)	Withdrawal of food and/or water, as defined by the project licence.

9)	Placement of avian eggs into previously set chillers at the termination of a procedure.'

A special proviso is applied, over and above the initial caveat demanding permission to delegate these non-technical procedures, in the case of the two final categories of non-technical procedures which a personal licensee can delegate. The following tasks can only be undertaken by assistants in the presence of a suitably authorised personal licensee.

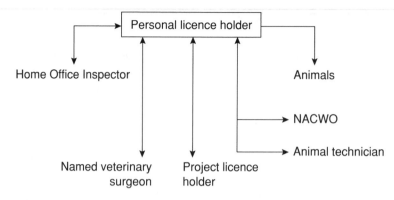

Fig. 6.1 Relationship of personal licence holder to other members of staff.

'10) In animals rendered insentient by decerebration or general anaesthesia which is to persist until death, and through an established catheter, administration of a substance(s) as defined by the project licence or removal of body fluids.

11) In animals rendered insentient by decerebration or general anaesthesia which is to persist until death, the administration of electric stimuli through electrodes implanted by a personal licensee.'

'During the performance of surgical procedures, unlicensed assistants may only perform the simplest of duties in the presence of, and in response to instructions from, the personal licence holder who is performing the procedure. Such duties may include the retraction of wound margins and the cutting of sutures or ligatures. Assistants without personal licence authorities may not make or close surgical incisions, or perform any other intervention requiring specific knowledge or technical skill.'

'The Home Office should be consulted if there is any doubt as to whether or not a regular procedure may be considered to be delegable. In all cases specific authority to delegate must be in the personal licence.'

(Guidance 6.26–27)

Figure 6.1 displays the various relationships of the personal licence holder to other members of staff involved with experimental animals.

Chapter 7

The Project Licence

Definition of 'project licence'

The official definition of a project licence is to be found in the Animals (Scientific Procedures) Act 1986.

> 's. 5(1) A project licence is a licence granted by the Secretary of State specifying a programme of work and authorising the application, as part of that programme, of specified regulated procedures to animals of specified description at a specified place or places.'

Salient features of the project licence are:

- authorisation of a programme including regulated procedures
- description of background, objectives and potential benefits of a project
- description of techniques entailed in each procedure
- statement of species and estimation of numbers of animals used
- the fixing of severity bands
- the naming of the establishment where the work is done
- statement of the name of the licensee and named deputies.

The licence itself and the application for it are issued to parties concerned when required so copies of them hardly belong within this text.

The application for a licence is by no means a simple matter. The process involved is more in the nature of making a case – justifying the performance of suggested procedures – rather than merely filling in an official questionnaire, or establishing appropriate qualifications, as may be required for the acquisition of other types of licence. The complicated nature of the application is well illustrated by the fact that time is set aside in the training of applicants for specific instruction in dealing with the application form. Special useful and illuminating seminars on this topic have been provided by the HO Inspectorate.

The Guidance Notes which accompany the form of application for a project licence contain indications on the type and form of information required by the inspector who considers the application initially. They have proved extremely helpful. In some designated establishments, dedicated staff are employed in the important area of liaison with the HO regarding project licences. They relieve the stress of the process for research workers. Some comment on the process of application would not be out of place.

Points worthy of note on the application for a project licence

The main source of difficulties in applying for a project licence is the fact that advocacy rather than form-filling is the theme of the exercise. Perhaps the most useful relevant accomplishment is rhetoric, in the best sense of the word. The applicant is expected to argue her/his case, and justify her/his project in the context of the cost/benefit assessment. A valuable hint is that a good legal counsel always asks 'Who is the judge going to be?', and they cut their cloth accordingly.

Good communication with the Inspector is crucial. Although published a while before the notes and examples associated with the application form of 2005 were published, seven points from past HO advice (November 2000) are worthy of repetition. Because your application is assessed in the first instance by your Inspector, consultation with her/him is highly recommended:

- To discuss format and content.
- Because Inspectors are experts in some areas of research and have access to a wide reservoir of expertise in the form of their colleagues (now standing at about 30) versed in other fields of research.
- To seek assistance about the wording of, description of, notification of, entry to, etc. regarding PODES.
- To seek advice about cases involving referral to the APC.
- To discuss re-use or continued use.
- To seek advice concerning severity bands.
- To seek advice on 'low maintenance authorities' i.e. avoiding inflexible details especially in protocol 19b.

Individual Inspectors may vary in their opinion on the appropriate ways of dealing with specific points within the application form. This is a topic which has come to the fore, with adverse comment, in the numerous 5th modules with which I have been involved in over the years. In mitigation, it may be said that a moderate flexibility is a desirable quality in the administration of law. Comparison of variable responses needs to take account of the fact that it is not always a matter of comparing like with like. The details of applications for project licences, in my own experience, may vary tremendously.

There is a new project licence form (2005), fully adapted to be completed electronically, except for the Declarations section, pp. 2 and 3 (these pages call for signatures). This application form is in my opinion an improved version and is accompanied by notes and examples. There are no longer the ominous blank sheets of ss. 17 (Why?), 18 (How? – descriptive) and 19 (What you are doing? – prescriptive). Directions are now sprinkled over these pages to aid the bemused. Any stakeholder can attain a copy of this form and the attached guidance notes with examples.

On p. 1 of the guidance notes there is an important statement as regards confidentiality.

'Information in this application which is not exempt from disclosure has to be provided to enquirers on request, but applicants should be aware that several exemptions may apply. In particular, there are exemptions for information whose disclosure could lead to an action for breach of confidence or is prohibited under section 24 of the Animals (Scientific Procedures) Act 1986 or where disclosure would prejudice commercial interests, or would compromise the health and safety of individuals. Information that is already available or intended for publication within a reasonable time is exempt, and this would include information in the project abstract. Much of the information provided in a project licence application but not in the abstract is likely to fall within the exemptions.'

A HO statement (22/04/05) is relevant.

'Up to the end of March (2005) we have received seventeen requests for information relating to the production and use of animals for experimentation and other scientific purposes. Of these, four were from journalists, eight from Non Governmental Organisations (NGOs), and five from members of the public. The information requested has included the contents of inspection reports, details of projected licences, names of individuals, companies and academic institutions licensed under the Act, and information about the importation of non-human primates to the UK.

To date we have answered 13 of these requests, providing some fairly basic, non-sensitive information. No information has been provided about individuals working under the Act. Also, in handling a request for information contained in five of the project licences for which abstracts have been published on the Home Office website, we concluded there was little additional information to disclose beyond what was already provided in the well-constructed abstracts.

From these early cases, it appears that the Freedom of Information Act provides adequate safeguards for the information we hold, although none of our decisions have yet been tested through the appeal processes available to applicants.'

The topic of confidentiality will be discussed further in Chapter 13.

From time to time the Secretary of State has announced specific policies for certain types of work for which special reporting procedures are required, for example, testing for skin corrosivity. If the project contains work listed in s. 16a, an appropriate condition will be added to the project licence.

A Home Office Guidance Note was issued in 2005 – Supplementary Guidance to Applicants for Projects that Generate and/or Maintain Genetically Modified Animals.

Advice given in the past as regards the presentation of objectives is still valid; 'Objectives should be SMARTER – Specific, Measurable, Achievable, Relevant, Timely and able to be Evaluated and Reviewed'.

The licence application and the 3Rs

Replacement, reduction and refinement are essentials in both the application for and the granting of a project licence. The whole subject of the 3Rs has dominated, and rightly so, the ethical discussion on animal experimentation.

The strict obligation to seek for more acceptable expressions of the 3Rs in practice is not only ethical, but is solidly grounded in the A(SP)A.

> 'The Secretary of State shall not grant a project licence unless he is satisfied that the applicant has given adequate consideration to the feasibility of achieving the purpose of the programme to be specified by means not involving the use of protected animals.'

> (s. 5(5))

The Guidance comments on the implementation of the 3Rs in practice in nn. 5.13–20. For example; 'the Secretary of State will review, and may recall and revise, licence authorities should suitable replacement, reduction and refinement alternatives become available during the lifetime of a project licence.'

Our domestic legal requirements in respect to the 3Rs fully implement European legislation on the matter.

> 'An experiment shall not be performed if another scientifically satisfactory method of obtaining the result sought, not entailing the use of an animal, is reasonably and practically available.'
>
> (Directive 86/609/EEC, Art 23)

Statements on the scientific validity of the Rat Skin Transcutaneous Electric Resistance (TER) Test and the EPISKIN test signed by Michael Balls, Head of ECVAM and Guy Corcelle, Head of DGXI/E/2, European Commission, Brussels were quickly approved, accepted and applied in the UK in an official letter by Steve Wilkes, head of the Animal Procedures Section (29/6/1998):

> 'The European centre for the Validation of Alternative Methods (ECVAM) has validated two replacement skin-corrosivity tests, rat skin TER and EPISKIN. Authority to use animals to test skin corrosivity will only be given if a regulatory requirement can be established. All those with existing authorities to use animals in such tests should only do so where the in vitro alternative can be demonstrated to be inadequate.'

The Home Office issued a comment on this development regarding specific alternatives.

'The EU Committee for Adaptation to Technical Progress agreed on 4 February 2000 that three in vitro tests should be added to Annex V of Directive 67/548/EEC on the Classification, Packaging and Labelling of Dangerous Substances. Two of the in vitro tests (TER and EPISKIN) are for skin corrosivity and the third test (3T3 NRA) relates to phototoxic potential.

The three non-animal test methods were published in the EU Official Journal on 8 June and on 20 June the European Commission informed member states that for the purposes of Directive 86/609/EEC the three tests are considered to be scientifically validated and to be reasonably and practicably available.

As you will recall, last year we established in relation to the LD50 (OECD Guideline 401) test that Section 5(5) of the Animals (Scientific Procedures) Act 1986 (as amended in September 1998) prohibits the licensing of tests for which there is a reasonably practicable, scientifically validated alternative which replaces animal use entirely, uses fewer animals or causes less suffering. We also established that the requirements of international regulators have no bearing on these decisions.

The same consideration applies in the current case and The Inspectorate has noted and is already taking account of the availability of the three in vitro tests in assessing new applications for licences for regulatory toxicology and safety testing for skin corrosivity and phototoxic potential. Existing licences will now also be reviewed and recalled for the removal of authorities for the animal-based tests. Exceptions to this approach will only be made where justified on specific scientific grounds. Where a scientific case exists for continuation of such authorities, a special condition will be added to restrict their use to that purpose.'

The endeavours of ECVAM are ongoing activities so more developments may be anticipated in this area. No doubt the Inspectorate will keep stakeholders informed.

On an official level, the Inter-Departmental Data Sharing Group promoted the reduction aspect of the 3Rs by its publication in 2000 of the Inter-Departmental Data Sharing Concordat. In 2002 the Inter-Departmental Group on the 3Rs, headed by the Home Office and including other government bodies such as the Department of Health and DEFRA, was formed as a successor to the Inter-Departmental Data Sharing Group.

According to the Home Office (cf. http://www.homeoffice.gov.uk/docs2/interdept3rs.html), the Concordat was a voluntary scheme which sought to promote opportunities for encouraging agencies, industry and other stakeholders to endorse the principle of data sharing and to extend its scope by looking to overcome the practical, legal, commercial and cultural barriers to its effective implementation. Under the Concordat, UK regulatory authorities pressed for agreement on behalf of the UK government for fuller provisions and procedures which would enable data sharing when negotiating, updating and transposing relevant European Directives and when taking part in other international harmonisation processes.

The text of the Concordat can be found at: http://www.homeoffice.gov.uk/docs/dataconcordat.html. Unfortunately the last updated page on this website was 11 June 2002. Progress, however, in this area is being made by The National Centre for the Replacement, Refinement and Reduction of Animals in Research (NC3Rs).

In a wider field, the International Conference on Harmonisation of Technical Requirements for Registration of Pharmaceuticals for Human Use (ICH) brings together the regulatory authorities of Europe, Japan and the United States and experts from the pharmaceutical industry in the three regions. Their efforts should lead to a reduction in the need for duplication in testing during the development of new medicines (cf. ibid., p. 208).

Duration of a project licence

A project licence is valid for five years but may be issued for a shorter term. It is not transferable.

> 'Project licences are issued to individuals. If a project licence holder wishes to relinquish responsibility for the programme of work, or is no longer able to ensure compliance with terms and conditions of the licence, a fresh application for a project licence must be made by a new applicant if the programme of work is to continue.
>
> In exceptional cases, where:
>
> - the licence has very recently been issued; and
> - the sole change related to the licence holder; and
> - the new applicant has equivalent knowledge, skill and resources available to the former licence holder; and
> - where no change is required, a licence based upon the earlier authorities may be issued to the new applicant with the same expiry, licence number, and conditions of issue as the original licence.'
>
> (Guidance 5.80–81)

In such cases and indeed in a case where a renewal of a licence is sought, an application for a new licence should be made well before the expiry date of the original licence.

Note condition 21 of the standard conditions on certificates of designation.

> 'The certificate holder shall notify the Secretary of State of the death of a project licence holder within seven days of it coming to his or her knowledge when unless the Secretary of State directs otherwise, the project licence shall continue in force for 28 days from the date of notification. The certificate holder will, during that period, assume responsibility for ensuring compliance with the terms and conditions of the project licence.'

The 1991 APC Report (p. 7, nn. 2.11 and 13) would be of interest to senior members of the scientific community.

'Where a project licence is granted to a person aged 70 or more this will be for 12 months only and will be reviewed at the end of this period. Particular attention will also be paid during inspections to the work of any licence holder aged 70 or more.

In future project licences, including new project licences for the continuation of previously authorized work, which are applied for by those aged 65 or more will only by granted for that period which takes the applicant up to his or her 70th birthday.'

This rider stemmed from the Feldberg affair in 1990. I have had the honour of having a Japanese septuagenarian (though younger than myself) as a delegate at modules 1, 2 and 3, to whom a personal licence was to be issued.

Justification – cost/benefit

Polemics concerning the justification for the use of animals in research within the context of the cost/benefit assessment has been continuous background music to the evolution of the administration of the A(SP)A. The requisite legal justification was intended to be arrived at by a careful weighing up of the relationship, the proportionality, between the cost (perhaps the term 'harm' would be preferable), that is, the possible suffering of the animal, and the desirable consequences which are the hoped-for results of the research being pursued. An interesting note relevant to cost/benefit occurs in the Final Report of the Sub-Group Ethical Review of the Technical Expert Working Group for the revision of Directive 86/609/EEC on the protection of animals used for experimental and other scientific purposes, p. 3 (02/12/03).

'(Note: Some countries use the expression 'cost/benefit' but working group members felt this could be confusing in translation and that harm-benefit was more explicit. We suggest this terminology is used by all the working groups.)'

There is, however, a statement on the front of this report: 'The views expressed in this report do not necessarily reflect those of the European Commission.'

Numerous early expositions of this topic were produced by leading scientists. For example, the article by D. G. Porter in *Nature*, 356, 12 March 1991, pp. 101–102 and the Decision Cube of Professor Bateson which can be found, along with other outlines of proposed methods to strike the desired balance, in *Ethics, Animals and Science*, Dolan, K., Blackwell Science, Oxford, 1999, pp. 218–243.

It would seem appropriate at this point to indicate the continuing evolution in the interpretation in practice of the A(SP)A. This useful feature of the legislation is well illustrated by the consideration given to this theme in the 1996 Annual Report of the Animal Procedures Committee (pp. 27–28).

'18. The submissions we received revealed that there is a considerable degree of interest in how the cost/benefit assessment is deployed under the 1986 Act. Some of the submissions from animal protection groups were explicitly critical that very few applications for licences apparently "failed" the cost/benefit assessment. This suggested to them that the analysis is not strictly applied, or that the Inspectorate colludes with licence applicants. We do not accept this conclusion or the premises on which it is based.

19. Some submissions to the review, both from animal protection groups and the user community, suggested that there was uncertainty about how the cost/benefit assessment operated in practice: what factors were examined in the assessment, how was cost evaluated, what kind of benefits were considered and how were costs and benefits weighed against each other? In other words, there are questions about the standard that is applied and about the method of its application.

20. These are issues that the statement on cost/benefit will explore. Our proposal is to discuss these matters with the Inspectorate so that this statement can be built upon and be a critique of existing Home Office practice. In the end, the statement will represent the view of the Animal Procedures Committee and not necessarily that of the Home Office. Among other things, it will situate the Home Office cost/benefit at the end of the chain of events that lead up to an application for a licence; and will examine whether the cost/benefit assessment functions more as a controlling standard than providing a pass/fail examination of applications. One of the effects of a controlling standard is to improve scientific design and ensure that alternatives are employed whenever possible.

21. As for the method of application, there was the recognition that the cost/benefit assessment would always involve, in the end, a value judgement (but not an arbitrary, personal judgement with which it is commonly confused). Judgements are based on interpretation of agreed rules and on previous judgements and are informed by the management processes whereby the Home Office achieves consistency – all features introducing a high degree of objectivity into the decision making process.

22. It is also proposed to examine examples of cases which involve high costs to animals and others which involve low benefits for humans, other animals or the environment. We will also need to consider work aimed at advancing knowledge where the benefits may only accrue some way into the future and are less easy to identify. These "case studies" will show the cost/benefit assessment operating at the margins of what is acceptable under the Act – the

assumption being that, if it operates effectively in these cases, it will do so in less marginal cases.'

This attempt at incipient casuistry by the APC was most timely and proved to be of great advantage to those involved both in the application and observance of the A(SP)A. Throughout the history of English law, case law has played a crucial role in legal interpretation.

The delicacy of the casuistry called for in the assessment of cost/benefit is well illustrated in the APC 1997 Report (pp. 13–14) comment on the (1997) report produced by the Advisory Group on the Ethics of Xenotransplantation (the Kennedy Committee).

> '96. . . . The Kennedy Committee ruled out the use of primates as source animals, but concluded that it would be justifiable, under a cost/benefit analysis, to use such animals in research, where the benefit for a large number of humans would flow from the use of a much smaller number of primates. The Kennedy Committee also concluded that the use of pigs as sources of organs may be acceptable, but that the acceptability lay in balancing the benefit to humans against the costs to the pig.

> 97. These were views of some significance when it came to our own consideration of applications to use animals in xenotransplantation research, most obviously in the sense that the Kennedy Committee's conclusions were based on a method of cost/benefit assessment which is comparable to our own. As the passages in this report on xenotransplantation reveal, we are particularly sensitive to the issues arising from the use of wild-caught baboons in such research.'

More notes on the cost/benefit assessment

(APC Report 1997 pp. 43–59)

> '2. The question of whether the benefits derived outweigh the costs is a starting point for many people when contemplating the issues surrounding the use of animals for experimental purposes.

> 3. It is not surprising, therefore, that a cost/benefit assessment is central to the provision of the Animals (Scientific Procedures) Act 1986 and to the framework which it establishes for the protection of animals. In some cases, it serves to prohibit certain experiments and, in all cases, it encourages an awareness of the welfare costs which experimentation may involve. It is a key element, then, in ensuring a responsible and critical use of animals in scientific procedures, and provides the backbone of the current regulatory regime.'

The following 1993 APC Report's quasi-algebraic portrayal of cost/benefit was, however simplistic, a worthwhile beginning:

$$\text{'(i)} \quad \text{Justification} = \frac{\text{Benefit}}{\text{Cost}}$$

$$\text{(ii)} \quad = \frac{\text{Importance of objectives} \times \text{Probability of achievement}}{\text{Cost to animals in suffering}}$$

$$\text{(iii)} \quad = \frac{\frac{\text{Background/Objectives}}{\text{potential benefits}} \times \text{Scientific quality}}{\text{Adverse effects} - \text{Coping strategies}}$$

$$\text{(iv)} \quad = \frac{\text{Section 17} \times \text{Section 18}}{\text{Section 19}} \text{ of PPL'}$$

'5. In giving attention to the issue of the cost/benefit assessment, we have not meant to suggest that it is always difficult to find a consensus about costs and benefits. If we think of cases as lying on a spectrum, at one end we shall find a band where the costs are plainly great and the benefits small and, at the other end, a band in which the benefits are great and the costs small. There are other cases, however, where things are more finely balanced, and where the necessary exercise of judgement will be more open to question.'

In the 1997 APC Report, the Chief Inspector expanded and advanced the notion of the cost/benefit assessment:

'1.2. The cost/benefit assessment is applied at the project licence level, and is a process rather than an event. It generally begins before a formal application is made and continues throughout the duration of the programme of work, rather than being applied only at the time authorities are granted or refused. An outline is given of how the Inspectorate both assesses new proposals and ensures the 3Rs are properly implemented.

2.3. The 1993 paper [produced by the Inspectorate and published in the APC 1993 Report] stated that the cost/benefit assessment is applied at the project licence level, and argued that factors regulated by other parts of the system did not form part of this consideration. This is one area where thinking has changed. Although no cost benefit assessment is conducted when advising on personal licence or certificate of designation applications, technical competence and standards of care and accommodation are now considered during the project licence cost/benefit assessment.

3.8. Although a considerable body of precedent and case law has been established which is applied to new applications, the framework for the cost/benefit assessment is not, and should not be, a static system. Assessments reflect precedent, but also accommodate developments in welfare, science, ethics, political thinking and informed public opinion.

4.4. Applications set the animal-based research in the context of other activities and collaborative work being performed to meet the stated objectives. Experimental design must be sound and clearly suited to meeting the stated objectives. Justification is required for the animal models to be used and the specific endpoints requested (reflecting both welfare and scientific outcomes). It must be clear that the cost has been minimised and the benefits maximised.

4.5. A considerable proportion of Inspectorate resources is devoted to ensuring that project licence applications cannot be further refined, and that authorities are drafted in such a way that projects are reviewed if progress is not made or if unexpected welfare problems occur.'

Moving on from the 1997 APC Report, the Guidance (Appendix I) has official material on the moot point of the fundamental features of the cost/benefit assessment. The cost/benefit assessment became so significant that, after much consultation, a special lengthy APC Report was published solely on the topic in 2003. A weighty publication by the Nuffield Council on Bioethics, *The Ethics of Research Involving Animals*, London, 2005 (http:www.nuffieldbioethics.org) endorsed the findings of this APC Report. The following quotation is from the Nuffield Council on Bioethics (p. 274).

'15.54 The cost/benefit assessment is at the heart of the regulation of research on animals in the UK. There is sometimes the view that the assessment is only being carried out by the Home Office, which "tells the researchers what to do" once it has decided on whether or not a licence application fulfils the criteria of the A(SP)A and is thus, from the regulators point of view, acceptable. The APC's 2003 Report "Review of cost/benefit assessment in the uses of animals in research" observed that this interpretation would be simplistic, since other individuals and committees are involved in assessing directly or indirectly the costs and benefits of a project. The APC therefore emphasised that:

"project licence holder and others involved in study design and initiation bear responsibility for clearly setting out the costs and benefits of their research and carrying out cost/benefit assessments of their work, including critical evaluation of the need for animal studies at all. The roles of other bodies such as the Home Office, ERP, and, where relevant APC, are to evaluate, advise, and in some cases, adjudicate the researcher's own cost/benefit assessments."

15.55 We welcome this clarification, which is compatible with our discussion about moral agency. As we have said, it would be wrong to perceive acting morally simply as following rules. Instead, active and continued scrutiny of the costs and benefits is required from all those involved, before, during and after research. This responsibility cannot be devolved to regulators, and, as the APC has emphasised, the system is not intended to function in this way.'

Details of the 2003 APC Review of cost/benefit assessment can be found at www.apc.gov.uk/index.htm and the favourable response in 2005 of Caroline Flint, the Home Office Minister, at www.homeoffice.gov.uk/comrace/animals/index.html. She emphasises that the cost/benefit assessment should be seen as a continuous process. In no way can the full balance of benefit and cost be performed adequately by mathematical calculations (cf. Guidance Appendix I, n. 12).

Likely benefits

Although the cost/benefit mantra puts the term 'cost' first, in the licence application form the consideration of benefit in s. 17 precedes the assessment of cost.

> '6. The likely benefit is primarily derived from the utility of the data or product to result from the programme of work, rather that the importance of the general area of study. Thus, although the long-term objective may be to find medical treatments, the benefit for the purposes of the cost/benefit assessment relates to the progress likely to result directly from the programme outlined in the project licence application.
>
> 7. Applications for regulatory toxicity and safety testing are generally premised on the need to facilitate scientifically sound regulatory decisions for the protection of man and the environment, rather than on the utility or benefit of the end product. The requirements of international regulators do not, in themselves, constitute sufficient benefit if alternative tests are available.
>
> 8. The Secretary of State must be of the opinion that the programme of work is likely to meet its stated objectives and that the scientific quality of the work cannot be further improved.'
>
> (Guidance, Appendix I)

Proposed benefits must be within the scope of the stipulated reasons for the granting of a project licence:

- control of disease, ill-health or abnormality
- physiological studies
- environmental protection
- advancement of biological or behavioural science
- education or training
- forensic enquiries
- breeding genetically modified animals or harmful mutants.
  (cf. European Convention (Art II) and A(SP)A (s. 5(3))

Disbenefits

The Chief Inspector writing in the 1997 APC Report draws attention to a feature of research not always given an airing.

'5.25 Potential disbenefits (that is, the potential misuse of the resulting information or technologies) may be recognised. The Inspectorate considers that potential disbenefit does not strictly speaking, form part of the cost/benefit assessment; but that when foreseen, it must nevertheless be clearly signalled in the advice offered to the Secretary of State to facilitate any necessary wider consultation and consideration.'

Perhaps the controversial areas of genetic manipulation or warfare research may fall within the shadow of this notion of disbenefit.

Likely cost (or 'harm')

'9. "Cost" is considered as the adverse welfare effects (pain, suffering, distress or lasting harm) likely to be experienced by the protected animals used during the course of study. As outlined in paragraphs 2.13–2.23 of this Guidance, these may be produced by acts of commission or omission; they may be immediate or delayed; and they may be a specific consequence of the procedures or the result of, for example, the care and husbandry systems.

10. Reduction, refinement and replacement strategies (the 3Rs described by Russell & Burch in their 1959 book, *The Principles of Humane Experimental Technique*) must be demonstrably implemented in the context of the proposed work. Minimising suffering, not simply reducing the number of animals used in the objective. The minimum number of animals of the lowest degree of neurophysiological sensitivity should be used in the mildest protocols required to meet the stated objectives [Sections 5(5) A(SP)A].'

(Guidance, Appendix I)

Both legislation and the Home Office administrative controls have set boundaries to the extent of harm to which an experimental animal can be exposed. Such limits have played a vital part in the evolution of the A(SP)A in practice.

- At the Act's inception it was announced that project licences for training to develop or maintain manual skills will only be issued for training of practising surgeons in microvascular techniques, when no alternatives are available.
- In the Act itself it is stipulated that:
  (1) Animals must not be subjected to severe pain, distress or suffering that cannot be alleviated [s. 10(2a)]. 'Severe', however is open to interpretation.
  (2) A neuromuscular blocking agent must not be used instead of an anaesthetic (s. 17(b)). A condition of the licence demands the permission of the Secretary of State for use of a neuromuscular blocking agent in experiments involving animals.
- In 1997 it was announced that licences would not be issued for:
  (1) Testing finished cosmetics products and substances intended for use as cosmetics ingredients.

(2)   Development or testing of alcohol or tobacco products (though the use of tobacco or alcohol as research tools can be considered and licensed in the context of investigation of disease or novel treatments). The licensing system does not seem to have, and rightly so, an absolute bottom line. It is essentially a case-by-case system with a stringent set of controls for the protection and welfare of the animal.

(3)   Development or testing of offensive weapons (but licences can still be granted for developing and testing means of protecting people or treating the effects of weapons).

(4)   The use of great apes (that is, chimpanzee, pigmy chimpanzee, gorilla and orang-utan).

(5)   The use of the ascites method of monoclonal antibody production unless exceptionally this method can be proved to be the only possible one.

- In 1999 the government announced that the LD50 test (OECD 401) will no longer be allowed in the UK, but the test can still be licensed on 'exceptional scientific grounds' (though the insistence of a foreign regulatory authority would not justify an exception to this rule).

The 1998 Amendment of A(SP)A and 'cost'

The amending of the Act, particularly s. 10, contributed to reducing possible harm to the experimental animal particularly in the area of welfare. Innovations included:

- the demand for anaesthesia in Schedule 2A
- special protection for endangered species and animals from the wild
- the release of animals
- provision for the preservation of animals after procedures
- need for trained animal care staff
- stricter control of the killing of animals
- special requirements on identification
- stipulations on the essentials of good husbandry.

Note that the impact on the care of the animal to avoid unnecessary suffering is the paramount aim of the Codes of Practice. This topic and the prospects of updating them in the light of European discussions on the application of European Directive 86/609/EEC is dealt with in Chapter 10.

Reduction of cost by best practice

The first appearance of the now 'in word' (or rather phrase) 'best practice', in the context of A(SP)A as part of the title of an official document is: *Home Office Guidance Note. Results of a Survey of Best Practice in Dog Accommodation and Care* (1999). The concept has been taken up with vigour by animal workers in research. The MRC

Centre for Best Practice for Animals in Research (CBPAR) was created by the Medical Research Council (MRC) in May 2001. The Centre develops and disseminates best practice guidance and expert advice to all those involved with animal use (cf. http://www.mrc.ac.uk/Animal_use_in_Research_Call.html).

The House of Lords Select Committee on Animals in Scientific Procedures (cf. Report on Session 2001–02, p. 39, 7.21) highly recommended this initiative of a Centre for Best Practice for Animals in Research set up by the MRC.

The APC refers to some of the factors of best practice in its *Report of the cost/benefit Working Group of the APC*, 2003, pp. 82–83.

> 'For example, there should already be widespread consensus that animal procedures involving methods that have been superseded by refined techniques should not be allowed under the Act, and that the same principle should apply to standards of husbandry and care.
>
> [. . .]
>
> It is also important to consider the particular needs of the particular animals involved, and to be sensitive to the likely effects of experiments on the individuals used.
>
> In addition, more explicit recognition within project licences of costs due to capture, confinement, transport, husbandry systems and general handling should help to ensure that strategies are put in place to minimise their adverse effects on animals.'

In the letter to Certificate Holders (22/04/05) the Home Office noted with approval a scheme introduced by LASA (with support from Pfizer Ltd) to promote best practice.

> 'The scheme offers opportunities principally for Named Persons, their deputies and others concerned with the day to day care and welfare of animals intended for and used for scientific purposes to visit other establishments. It is intended to provide a mechanism for the identification and dissemination of technical refinements, improvements in experimental design and enhancements of husbandry procedures that promote the refinement of animal use, care and husbandry.'

The previous sentence is an ideal description of the connotation of 'best practice' (cf. http://www.lasa.co.uk/bursaries/goodpractice.asp or email LASA@btconnect .com).

The grading of 'cost' – protocol severity limits

The Guidance covers this vital topic in nn. 5.40–49 (pp. 32–33). The wording used is well chosen and needs to be studied carefully in order that what is demanded in practice may be fully understood.

'The severity limit for each protocol is determined by the upper limit of the expected adverse effects that may be encountered by a protected animal, taking into account the measures specified in the licence for avoiding and controlling adverse effects. It represents the worse potential outcome for any animal subjected to the protocol, even if it may only be experienced by a small number of the animals to be used.

In assessing the severity of a protocol, account should be taken of the effect of all the procedures (whether regulated or not) applied to each animal or group of animals; the nature and extent of the likely adverse effects; the action taken to mitigate these effects; and the humane endpoints to be applied.

The severity limits of the protocols in the licence are categorized as follows:

- *Unclassified*
  Protocols performed entirely under general anaesthesia, from which the animal does not recover consciousness. This includes the preparation and use of decerebrated animals.

- *Mild*
  Protocols that, at worse, give rise to slight or transitory minor adverse effects. Examples include, small infrequent blood samples; skin irritation tests with substances expected to be non-irritant or mildly irritant; minor surgical procedures under anaesthesia such as small superficial tissue biopsies or cannulation of peripheral blood vessels. However, if used in combination or repeated in the same animal the cumulative severity may be increased beyond mild. Protocols may also be regarded as mild if they have the potential to cause greater suffering but contain effective safe-guards to initiate effective symptomatic or specific treatment or terminate the protocol before the animal shows more than minor adverse effects.

- *Moderate*
  Protocols regarded as moderate include toxicity tests (which do not include lethal endpoints) and many surgical procedures (provided that suffering is controlled and minimised by effective post operative analgesia and care). Protocols that have the potential to cause greater suffering, but include controls which minimise severity or terminate the protocol before the animal shows more than moderate adverse effects, may also be classed within the moderate severity limit.

- *Substantial*
  Protocols that may result in a major departure from the animal's usual state of health or well-being. These include: acute toxicity procedures where significant morbidity or death is an endpoint; some efficacy tests of anti-microbial agents and vaccines; major surgery; and some models of disease, where welfare may be seriously compromised. If it is expected that even one animal would suffer substantial effects, the procedure would merit "substantial" severity limit.

The Secretary of State will not licence any procedure likely to cause severe pain or distress that cannot be alleviated [section 10(2A)].'

The severity condition

'Licence holders are required by conditions in both project and personal licences to minimise any pain, suffering, distress or lasting harm. They should approach the limit of severity which has been authorized only when absolutely necessary to meet the specific objective [Sections 10(2) and 5(5)].'

(Guidance 5.43)

'If it seems likely that the severity limit of a procedure has or may be exceeded, the project licence holder, or deputy licence holder, must contact the Home Office. Provided the project licence holder can show sufficient justification, the Secretary of State may temporarily authorize a higher severity limit for a period of up to 14 days to allow the balance of likely benefit and likely cost to be reviewed and amendment to the project licence to be considered.'

(Guidance 5.44)

'The project licence condition will be regarded as breached if the Home Office is not notified promptly by the project licence holder (or deputy) when a protected animal has, as the result of the regulated procedures performed suffered (or is likely to suffer) more than is authorized by the severity limit. It will also be regarded as breached if the endpoints applied resulted in more suffering than was necessary to achieve the specific objectives.'

(Guidance 5.45)

'The condition may be considered to have not been breached if the suffering arose from an unforeseeable, extraneous reason (that is, a problem unrelated to the regulated procedures), providing adequate and effective steps have been taken promptly to alleviate the suffering.'

(Guidance 5.46)

The overall severity band of a project (Guidance 5.47–49)

'The assessment of the overall severity of a project will reflect the cumulative effect of each procedure. This assessment is used by the Secretary of State to weigh the likely adverse effects on all the animals to be used against the benefits likely to accrue.'

(cf. A(SP)A s. 5(4))

The assessment of the severity band for the project reflects the number of animals used on each protocol and the actual suffering likely to be caused as a result. It is based on the overall level of cumulative suffering to be experienced by each animal, not just the worst possible case. It takes into account the proportion of animals expected to reach the severity limit of the protocol and the duration of the

Table 7.1   Project licences

Severity band	In force on 31 December 2004		Granted during 2004		Revoked during 2004	
	Number	%	Number	%	Number	%
Mild	1116	38	214	37	254	40
Moderate	1641	56	334	58	346	54
Substantial	56	2	12	2	14	2
Unclassified	86	3	15	3	20	3
Total	2899		575		634	

From 'Statistics of Scientific Procedures on Living Animals in Great Britain in 2004', London, HMSO (Cm. 67813), (2005). Available on the Home Office Science and Research website: www.homeoffice.gov.uk/science-research/

exposure to that severity limit, the nature and intensity of the adverse effects, and the actions to be taken to relieve the suffering.

The assessment of severity (of individual protocols or the project as a whole) should be reviewed and revised as necessary during the lifetime of a project. This ongoing review of projects is an important function of the Local Ethical Review Process which has been fully commented upon in Guidance Notes on Retrospective Review, a Discussion Document prepared by the LASA Ethics and Training Group (editors Maggy Jennings and Bryan Howard, December 2004) (cf. www.lasa.co.uk).

The Home Office Minister, Caroline Flint, invited the APC (02/10/03) to consider the issue of severity bands and limits, with a view to providing practical recommendations for a new system. As yet (in 2007) there are no official details concerning the fulfilment of this proposal. No doubt they will appear in due season.

Table 7.1 details the number of project licences which were active on 31 December 2004, the number granted during 2004 and the number revoked during 2004 (normally either at the licence holder's request or because the licence had run the maximum allowed term of five years). The total figures are subdivided into severity bandings.

Humane endpoints

'The Secretary of State must be satisfied that the protocols incorporate best practice and will be applied competently. Project licence applicants are required to provide a full description of measures proposed to prevent or minimise the extent, duration and incidence of the adverse effects. These may include the specification of humane endpoints and control measures (such as inspection schedules, the criteria used to assess the adverse effects, and the means to be used to minimise them).'

(Guidance 5.18)

'Humane endpoints should be set to provide for a number of eventualities: the research objectives having been achieved; the realisation that they cannot be achieved; or when welfare problems are encountered which exceed the minimum necessary to achieve the objective.'

(Guidance 5.19)

The severity of a procedure may be reduced by the use of appropriate end-points. Project licence applications involving procedures which may have specific adverse effects should wherever possible specify the action which will be taken in order to mitigate these effects. This could include withdrawing the animal from the procedure or humane killing.

In practice, humane endpoints may vary greatly from, for example, geriatric status as regards some non-human primates in defined cases to much more specific conditions as illustrated in a relevant publication on this matter.

'3.1 Considerable care should be given to the judicious choice of endpoint for tumour growth. This should take into account predictable indications of pain, distress or significant deviation from normal behaviour. Unless specified otherwise on the project licence, animals should be killed before:
1. predictable death occurs;
2. they get into poor condition;
3. the tumour mass becomes over-large, likely to ulcerate or unacceptably limits normal behaviour.'

'3.10 Humane endpoints and other procedures should be refined in the light of experience.'

(UKCCCR Guidelines for the Welfare of Animals in Experimental Neoplasia, 1988 (UKCCCR, 20 Park Crescent, London W1N 4AL))

The managerial role of the project licence holder

Supervision is among the most onerous duties of the project licence holder. The project licence holder, unfairly perhaps, and even unrealistically in some circumstances, may be deemed to be aware of all occurrences within her/his programme of research. He/she may, consequently, be liable to sanctions for misdemeanours committed by others within her/his project. Particularly important in this context is condition 14 requiring supervision of personal licences.

Besides the attention to the overall control of the project the project licence holder should take cognisance of:

(a) the provision of requisite facilities
(b) proper animal care
(c) observance in full of all the conditions on the licence
(d) the need for permission to move, transfer (between projects) or release animals included in the project

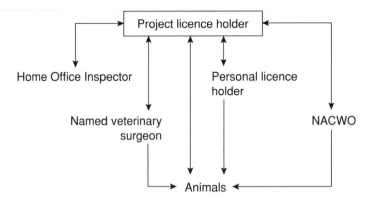

Fig. 7.1 Relationship of project licence holder with other interested parties.

(e) the obligation legally to conduct the project under the terms of the Act
(f) the duty to keep the programme within the permitted purpose stated in the application
(g) the limit set on the species and number of animals to be used
(h) the need for personal licensees to have authority for the regulated procedures they perform
(i) the awareness of and compliance with the severity conditions on the part of all licensees working within the project licence
(j) the appropriate training and guidance of personal licensees involved in the project
(k) the requirement for full and accurate records
(l) the obligation on personal licensees to ensure all animals are identified.

The deputy project licence holder

It is indicative of the importance of the managerial role of the project licence holder that special significance is given to the need for deputy licence holders. This is particularly the case if there could be a lacuna or gap in the impact of management on any area of the research programme.

The scope of the authority assigned to the deputy will vary. In some cases it may be appropriate, for example, for the project licence holder to delegate to the deputy the power to sign on his/her behalf documents pertinent to the project.

It is apparent from the wide responsibilities associated with a project licence that it is usually advisable that the project licence holder have a deputy or deputies since joint project licences are unacceptable. In some circumstances a deputy project licence holder must be appointed:

(i) where the nature or scope of the project is such that control is best exercised through one or more deputy project licence holders;
(ii) where work is to be done at more than one place so that a deputy is available locally to supervise the work on the project licence holder's behalf;

(iii)   where the project licence holder is likely to be absent for more than a month at a time;

(iv)   where the project licence holder does not hold a personal licence, in which case at least one deputy who holds a personal licence is required.

The deputy licence holder must be in a position to exercise day-to-day control over the work and to cover for the project licence holder's absence. His or her identity must be made known to those working on the project. A deputy licence holder will normally hold, or have held, a personal licence.

Project licence holders remain accountable for the performance and conduct of their deputies. The new project licence application form (2005) gives prominence to the role of the deputy licence holder by demanding their signature in the Declarations section.

Amendments to licences

Amendments to licences may be needed when:

- material discrepancies occur between predicted and adverse effects
- new objectives are added
- new or revised protocols are to be introduced to assist in meeting the objectives or to incorporate new 3Rs strategies
- estimated numbers need revision
- details of licence holder or deputies need updating
- availabilities need to be added or deleted.

Requests to the Home Office for amendments must have gone through the ethical review process and been signed by the Certificate Holder.

The Guidance 5.76 stresses that:

'Licence amendments do not take effect until the revised authorities have been issued by the Home Office. Project licensees must not anticipate revised authorities; they should await receipt of the amended licence documents; make sure that they and the personal licence holders are familiar with the terms and conditions of the amended authorities; and supply a copy of the revised authorities to the certificate holder. (When a project licence allows work at a "secondary availability" the licensee must copy these authorities to the second certificate holder before procedures are carried out.)'

The facility for amendment of licences and certificates and the ready availability of the process is one of the beneficial effects of the flexibility of the administration of the A(SP)A. Liaison with the Inspector is always useful and instructive in any negotiations as regards licenses but is particularly valuable when applying for an amendment.

Chapter 8

Training of Those with Responsibilities Under the A(SP)A

The five modules

The introduction of mandatory education and training of project and personal licence holders appeared in the 1992 APC Report.

'n. 6.3. From 1 April 1994 applicants for personal licences will be required to have completed successfully an accredited training programme. In addition to this, from 1 April 1995, those project licence applicants seeking a project licence for the first time will require further pre-licence training to be acquired from accredited training programmes . . . All training programmes for applicants for personal and project licences are to be accredited under a scheme recognised by the Home Office.'

In practice this training takes the form of five modules:

Module 1 Elements
(1)   Historical background
(2)   An introduction to ethical aspects of the use of animals in scientific procedures
(3)   The Animals (Scientific Procedures) Act 1986
(4)   Other relevant legislation

Module 2 Elements
(1)   Recognition of well-being, pain, suffering or distress
(2)   Handling and restraint
(3)   Humane methods of killing
(4)   Local procedures
(5)   Personal health and safety

Modules 3 Elements
(1)   Biology and husbandry
(2)   Common diseases and recognition
(3)   Health monitoring and disease prevention or control
(4)   Introduction to anaesthesia and analgesia
(5)   Conduct of minor procedures

Module 4 Elements
(1) Surgical anaesthesia and analgesia
(2) Conduct of surgical procedures

Module 5 Elements
(1) Ethical aspects of the use of live animals
(2) Analysis of the literature
(3) Alternatives
(4) Project design
(5) Project licence management
(6) Legal aspects – the European and wider international context.

An applicant for a personal licence is required to complete an accredited training programme including modules 1, 2 and 3 and also module 4 where appropriate (see Table 8.1 for more detail).

Table 8.1   Training of personnel under the A(SP)A

Target audience	Modules				
	1	2	3	4	5
Those not applying for a licence Personnel with administrative responsibilities only	★				
Non-licensed animal users; those killing by a schedule 1 method	★	★			
Licence applicants Undergraduates applying for limited personal licences to work under close supervision	★	★			
Personal licence applicants who will be performing minor non-surgical procedures; brief terminal procedures under anaesthesia	★	★	★		
Personal licence applicants who will be performing major surgical procedures under terminal or recovery anaesthesia	★	★	★	★	
Project licence applicants	★	★	if apt		★

The training requirements of former personal licensees who are applying for reinstatement of their licences will be determined by many factors including previous formal training and the length of time away from the use of animals in procedures. In such circumstances the person involved should discuss the matter with the Inspector. Personal licensees seeking significant amendments to the species authorised on the licence which involve additional skills (e.g. extension from rodent to dogs or to farm animals) will be expected to undergo additional practical training for such amendment.

New applicants for project licences are required to have successfully completed at least modules 1, 2 and 5 and also modules 3 and 4 when appropriate to the procedures in the project.

Exemptions from mandatory training requirements

Appendix B of the 1992 APC Report states:

> 'All exemptions are discretionary on a case-by-case basis and should be discussed with the Inspector before application for a licence is made. The following examples indicate the types of circumstances in which exemptions will be considered.'

Personal licence applicants

> 'Exemption from all training requirements will be considered only for those persons with formal training in laboratory animal science, for example holders of a Certificate or Diploma in Laboratory Animal Science of the Royal College of Veterinary Surgeons, the MSc in Laboratory Animal Science of the University of London or the Associateship [now the Membership] or Fellowship of the Institute of Animal Technology.
>   Completion of module 1 only will be considered:

- for applicants for personal licences valid only for practical work on a micro-surgery training course, the licence to be surrendered immediately upon completion of the course. The contents of this module may be incorporated into the micro-surgery course itself;
- for veterinary surgeons with practical experience of the relevant species;
- for animal technicians highly experienced with the relevant species;
- for holders of qualifications in laboratory science from outside the UK. They will be expected to complete module 1 to ensure familiarity with UK law.

Completion of modules 1 and 2 only will be considered:

- for applicants for very limited species and techniques (e.g. one species, oral dosing only);
- for undergraduates who will be under close supervision and with limited authorities; the contents of these modules may be integrated into the undergraduate course;
- for experienced overseas researchers.

Completion of modules 1 and 3 only will be considered:

- for applicants with extensive experience of the relevant species.'

Other Home Office requirements regarding training

'It is strongly recommended that deputy project licence holders successfully complete module 5.'

(Guidance 2.80)

The APC recommended that the training of NACWOs should be mandatory and produced a draft syllabus which would entail a minimum of 12 hours' course attendance/private study, excluding assessment time (attendance on Home Office module 1 – could be taken into consideration).

As from the middle of 2004 new Named Animal Care and Welfare Officers have been required to undertake training. The training consists of a syllabus proposed by the Institute of Animal Technicians (www.iat.org.uk). The same Institute is the Accrediting Body for these introductory NACWO courses as well as the Higher Education Staff Development Agency (HESDA) (www. Hesda.org.uk).

A Home Office Circular of 27 August 2004 informed certificate holders that introductory training for new NACWOs was mandatory.

By the end of 2005 Bioscientific Events Ltd (www.bioscientific.co.uk), a leading company in this field of training, had already trained 400 NACWOs.

The Home Office requires new Named Veterinary Surgeons to take a course approved and monitored by the Royal College of Veterinary Surgeons. Over and above this basic requirement the Royal College of Veterinary Surgeons encourages further provision of training in this field. The Home Office will consider exemptions from specific training where appropriate (cf. Guidance 2.77).

The Home Office advises applicants for certificates of designation to complete module 1 training. Certificate Holders as a group instigate further awareness exercises of their role among themselves through a Certificate Holders Forum (cf. Guidance 2.79).

Information on this topic can be found at http://www.homeoffice.gov.uk/comrace/animals.index.html

A private note: An obvious flaw in the efficient implementation of these very worthy schemes for the enlightenment of those involved arises from the fact that frequently intermingled with extremely fluent and highly educated scientists there are equally highly educated and intellectual research workers who find real difficulty in understanding English, not only in dealing with legal matters but even in ordinary parlance. They are sometimes more experienced and more highly qualified than some of the native delegates present. Having encountered this contretemps on more than a once-monthly basis for the last 12 years, I plead with the APC to seriously consider the problem.

The topic of training associated with the issue of licences and work with animals in research is fluid. There are at present (in 2007) proposals to remodel existing systems. It is suggested that modules 1 to 4 should be replaced with certain adjustments by modules A to E. Such amendments are bound to crop up from time to time as the years go by (cf. LASA *The Forum*, No. 3, Vol. 2, 2005). The website www.lasa.co.uk could prove useful for monitoring future changes.

Note: A Federation of European Laboratory Animal Sciences Associations booklet entitled *Laboratory Animals* gives details of the European-accepted accredited training for all engaged in the use of live vertebrate animals for scientific purposes. Evidence of this training, to FELASA recommended standards, is acceptable to the Home Office when combined with completion of module 1 of the UK mandatory training.

Chapter 9

Certificates of Designation

Designated establishments

Every regulated procedure must be performed within the provisions of a project licence, a personal licence and a certificate of designation. The requisite authorisation for the use of experimental animals may be indicated thus:

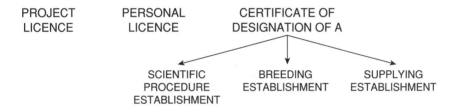

The interdependence and interlocking of the two forms of licences have already been discussed. The three forms of certificates are, however, discrete; one in no way depends upon the other, they exist separately and various establishments may have only one or all three.

Section 7 of the Act legislates in a similar manner to s. 6 for breeding and supplying establishments, for example, requiring the naming of the three responsible persons. The earliest edition of Home Office Guidance Notes (Question 3, p. 3) defined each type of establishment in reference to its function:

> 'User establishments will include premises where animals are held, before, during and after procedures, but not bred. These will need certificates of designation as scientific procedure establishments.
>
> If animals are bred for use in the same establishment or somewhere else, the premises where they are bred will need certificates of designation as breeding establishments.
>
> If animals are kept at an establishment where they have not been bred, for supply elsewhere, the premises will need certificates of designation as supplying establishments.'

Establishments which qualify for more than one of the certificates must apply for each designation which is appropriate. An establishment which breeds animals with harmful genetic mutations or genetically manipulated animals or supplies surgically prepared animals must also be designated as a scientific procedure establishment.

PODEs

Section 6(2) of A(SP)A allows for exceptional cases. A place specified in the personal and the project licence may be a place other than a designated scientific procedure establishment. There is information on this in the Guidance:

'2.66 The Secretary of State may grant such authority if it is inappropriate to designate the place – for example, where procedures must take place at a field site. Such authorities are coupled to additional project licence conditions that require the licensee to notify the Home Office prior to any procedure being performed. This allows a Home Office inspector to be present when the work is carried out. Additional safeguards are also applied to ensure the welfare of any animals that are to be left unattended or released to the wild following a regulated procedure (see paragraphs 5.51–5.54).'

Further details can be found in the Guidance Notes to the Application for a project licence on p. 4, No. 13.

'You must specifically justify any request to perform regulated procedures at any Place Other than a Designated Establishment ("PODE" site).

In addition to sites for work in the wild, PODE sites may include farms, health-screening laboratories and slaughterhouses where scientific data is to be obtained from the carcase.

Additional controls will apply (including notification conditions and requirements for certification of fitness of animals to be left unattended after the performance of regulated procedures).

Seek advice from an inspector on the precise wording to describe the non-designated sites, and the likely notification requirements. Notification conditions are intended to allow the Inspectorate to scrutinise work in progress.

Explain and justify, at section 18 of the application, why it is necessary to perform work at the PODE sites. Set out the systems proposed to ensure that animals will be certified fit by a competent person before being left unattended or released after or during the course of the regulated procedures. Demonstrate that the use of PODE sites poses no public health or environmental risk. Appropriate details should also be given in sections 19b(v).

It is your responsibility to ensure that any other relevant legislative requirements are identified and fulfilled (e.g. that any necessary authorities under the Wildlife and Countryside Act etc, are sought and obtained).

Ensure that, if appropriate, the landowner's consent has been secured prior to the application being submitted to the Home Office for assessment, and

Table 9.1 Certificates of Designation

Establishment type	In force on 31/12/2004	Granted during 2004	Revoked during 2004
Commercial concern	82	0	3
Higher education	84	2	1
Quango	30	0	1
Government	10	0	1
Non-profit	13	0	0
NHS hospital	5	0	0
Public health	3	0	0
Total	227	2	6

From 'Statistics of Scientific Procedures on Living Animals in Great Britain in 2004', London, HMSO (Cm. 67813) (2005). Available on the Home Office Science and Research website: www.homeoffice.gov.uk/science-research/

confirm that access to the site by Home Office inspectors for the purpose of inspecting licensed work has been facilitated.'

Table 9.1 details the number of certificates of designation which were in force on 31 December 2004, the number granted during 2004 and the number revoked during 2004. The figures are subdivided for different types of establishment.

Nominated persons

On every certificate of designation at least three persons must be nominated – the certificate holder (CH), the named animal care and welfare officer(s) (NACWO) and the named veterinary surgeon(s) (NVS).

Under s. 6(5) of A(SP)A there is an obligation on every applicant for a certificate of designation to appoint one or more persons as named animal care and welfare officers and named veterinary surgeons.

I have encountered numerous animal carers who have been concerned that they have various roles as regards the animals and they worry, as animal technicians are wont to do, about the possible conflict of interests. The Guidance is both clear and helpful in this matter.

'The contractual relationships between and other responsibilities of, these individuals can create conflicts of interest. There may also be occasions when one individual legitimately fulfils more than one of these roles. For example, in most cases, project licence holders, will hold or will have held, a personal licence. For these reasons, the Secretary of State normally requires that, for any group of protected animals, at least three individuals should fill these roles.'

(n. 3.18)

These five roles are certificate holder, project licence holder, personal licence holder, named veterinary surgeon and named animal care and welfare officer.

> 'When a named veterinary surgeon or named animal care and welfare officer has (under any other of the statutory roles) a substantial interest in the scientific outcome of a programme of work, alternative provision should be made for the veterinary or welfare oversight of the animals in question.'
>
> (n. 3.19)

Section 7 and Schedule 2 of the A(SP)A

Section 7 of A(SP)A regulates breeding and supplying establishments:

> 's. 7. (1) A person shall not at any place breed for use in regulated procedures (whether there or elsewhere) protected animals of a description specified in Schedule 2 of this Act unless that place is designated by a certificate issued by the Secretary of State under this section as a breeding establishment.'

and

> '(2) A person shall not at any place keep any such protected animals which have not been bred there but are to be supplied for use elsewhere in regulated procedures unless that place is designated by a certificate issued by the Secretary of State under this section as a supplying establishment.'

Under Schedule 2 animals may be obtained only from a designated supplying establishment. If a scientific procedure establishment does not breed its own animals (if it does, it would presumably already be designated as a breeding establishment), the animals listed below must be obtained only from a designated breeding establishment:

Dog
Cat

The animals listed below must be obtained from a designated breeding or supplying establishment:

Mouse
Rat
Guinea-pig
Hamster
Rabbit
Quail*
Non-human primates

Added to this second list from 1/1/1999 were:

Ferret
Gerbil
Genetically modified pig
Genetically modified sheep

⋆ This restriction only applies to *Coturnix coturnix*, the European Quail, and not, for example, to *Coturnix japonica*.

Consequences of Schedule 2

An overseas breeding or supplying establishment cannot be certified under the Act. Consequently, consent is required for the use of all imported cats and dogs, and also for the use of imported Schedule 2 species unless they have been acquired from a supplying establishment. The Secretary of State can grant an exemption from the demands of Schedule 2 (Code of Practice for the Housing and Care of Animals used in Scientific Procedures (later referred to as CODHCASP) 3.5).

Since 1996 primates can be acquired from overseas breeding centres only if these centres have been approved by the Home Office (APC Report 1997, p. 78, n. 4).

While there is no restriction in the A(SP)A on importation as such, one should seek Home Office approval to ensure that animals may be used once they have been imported.

> 'Details about licences, health certificates, rabies and other quarantine requirements should be obtained from the Animal Health Division, DEFRA.'

Cessation and amendment of certificates

Certificates remain in force until revoked. They may be revoked at the request of the certificate holder or by the Secretary of State if there is a breach of a condition or in other cases when the Secretary of State considers it appropriate to do so. Revocation might be appropriate if there is serious or persistent non-compliance with the conditions, failure to pay the fees or where the named persons are not able to meet their responsibilities and replacements (with the necessary amendments) have not been sought. Revocation immediately invalidates all personal and project licence 'availabilities' and animals may no longer be bred, kept for use, or used on regulated procedures at that establishment.

A certificate holder may request an amendment of the certificate at any time. Amendments are needed if there are changes in the title of the establishment, the class of designation, the persons named on the certificate, the list of the approved areas or the ethical review process. The new authorities are not valid until a revised certificate is issued by the Home Office (cf. Guidance 4.70–75).

The certificate holder (CH)

The role of this nominated person has evolved, in my experience, from in some cases being a distant cipher, far removed from the animal house – for example, the vice-chancellor of a university, or the bursar of an institution performing the primary legal obligation of paying the fees (cf. s. 8 of the A(SP)A) – to being a pivotal figure in the hands-on management of an animal facility.

The CH assumes responsibility for compliance with the terms and conditions on the certificate and any additional conditions imposed by the Secretary of State. Consequently the CH should have sufficient authority within the establishment to be able to properly discharge all their responsibilities under the A(SP)A. The Guidance reflects the importance of the fulfilment of these responsibilities by devoting more than four pages to the topic. The responsibilities are grouped under eight headings and can be studied in detail in the Guidance (nn. 4, 12–47).

1. The CH is responsible for taking all reasonable steps to prevent the performance of unauthorised procedures. The CH must see that systems of management and clear lines of communication are established to all interested parties, particularly with a view to avoiding any possible conflict of interest. The CH must ensure that licensees seek and take the appropriate advice from the NACWO and NVS.
2. The CH has an overall responsibility for the care and accommodation of the animals and so must ensure that:
   - areas are used as specified;
   - the fabric and environment of the approved areas are in keeping with the Code of Practice;
   - the appropriate environment, space, food, water and care for the animals are available;
   - restrictions on the animals are minimal;
   - the conditions in which the animals are kept will be checked daily and any deficiency will be attended to without delay;
   - the well-being of the animals are monitored daily to prevent unnecessary suffering;
   - if necessary, quarantine and acclimatisation facilities are available;
   - fire precautions and security measures against intruders and to prevent the escape of the animals are in place. Usually the named persons, the NACWO and NVS, will be more directly responsible for the above commitments but the CH must see that they discharge their duties and should supply all the documentation and information relevant to their work.
3. The CH should ensure that the following factors essential to the running of an animal facility, in keeping with legal requirements are in place:
   - provision of reasonable access for the Inspector to all parts of the establishment;
   - notification to the Inspector of any changes to named persons or use of rooms within the designated establishment;

- efficient discharge of their duties by the NACWO(s) and NVS;
- appropriate staffing and training of licensees;
- availability of competent persons to kill animals humanely and a list of such personnel;
- acquisition of animals from appropriate sources;
- issue of animals to authorised persons only;
- proper identification of all primates, dogs and cats by a method agreed with the Inspector;
- records of source, use and disposal of animals are kept;
- proper functioning of the LERP which implies, for example, confirmation by the CH's signature that each PPL application has completed the LERP and that all suitable facilities will be made available.

Figure 9.1, from the Guidance (p. 15), illustrates the relationships between the CH and other persons associated with a designated establishment.

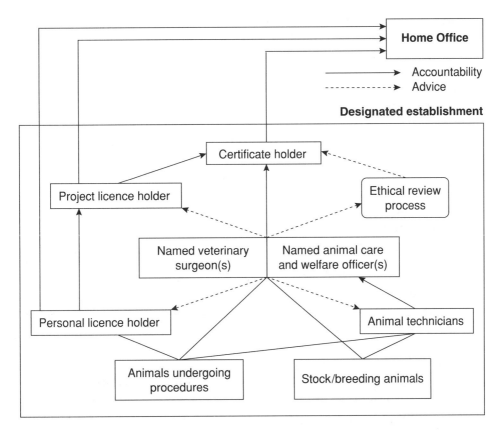

Fig. 9.1 Relationships within a designated establishment. Note: the advisory roles have been simplified in this diagram.

The local ethical review process (LERP)

The history of the A(SP)A as an enabling Act portrays a tendency for recommendations and even suggestions, especially from the APC, to become closely associated with and sometimes imperceptibly to pass into legislation. In keeping with a suggestion by the APC, the Home Secretary suggested the introduction of a Local Ethical Review Process in all Designated Establishments (Home Office PCD Circular 2/96 ref. 80/7801). By April 1999 the requirement for an LERP was a standard condition (condition 20 or 23, according to the type of certificate) on every certificate of designation.

The LERP should ensure as wide an involvement of the staff of the establishment as possible to consider both the application of the 3Rs and the welfare of the animals kept there. Appendix J of the Guidance presents the main features of the LERP.

- *Aims* – Provision of independent ethical advice to the CH especially as regards project licence applications and animal care. Although much of the discussion concerning LERPs tends to be concerned with project licence applications and the 3Rs, the fact that both breeding and supplying establishments, where there may be no project licences, must have an LERP, is a clear indication that the review process must be seriously concerned with animal welfare and other related animal matters. Relevant related matters are, for example, amendments to licences, retrospective reviews, cost/benefit assessment, humane killing procedures, provision of relevant information, provision of a forum for wide discussion on animal use, review of managerial systems and the provision of appropriate training for all those dealing with the animals. On the difficult topic of retrospective reviews of licences, useful Guidance Notes were produced by the LASA Ethics and Training Group, edited by Maggy Jennings and Bryan Howard, in December 2004.
- Provision of support and advice to named persons and licensees as regards both ethical issues and animal welfare.
- Promotion of ethical analysis to increase awareness of welfare issues and increase the application of the 3Rs.
- *Responsibility of the CH* – The CH appoints the people to be involved in the process, particularly the members of an associated committee which normally crystallises from the process and encapsulates the end result. The CH is fully responsible for the operation of the LERP.
- *Personnel* – The NVS and the NACWO must be involved in the process since a project licensee applicant must vouch on the application form that they have consulted both these officials concerning their application. Project and personal licensees should be represented in the process. The HO encourages the involvement of as many people as possible in the LERP, particularly those who do not have any responsibilities under the Act. It is recommended that one or more lay (an ambiguous term) persons independent of the establishment might be brought into the process. As yet it is not mandatory to have a statistician in the LERP though their services would emphasise the role of

'reduction' in the application of the principle of the 3Rs. The inspector may attend meetings of an ethical committee. Records of the ethical process, however, must be readily available to the inspector if requested.

- *Operation* – There should be regular deliberations and records of discussions and advice. Named persons and licensees should be kept informed of the progress of the LERP and encouraged to draw relevant matters to its attention. Input should be welcomed from stakeholders and all interested parties.

Inspectors are still happy to discuss early ideas with prospective project licence holders and will be available for advice and clarification. Only when the licence application has been signed by the CH, which is taken as proof that the application has been through the LERP, will it be considered for the formal authorisation by the HO. The inspector will not negotiate with any advisory group (cf. Guidance, Appendix J).

The evolution of the LERP in practice has been stimulated by numerous workshops on the topic. The ambience in which they have operated – whether, for example, they are set in a pharmaceutical company or an academic environment – has influenced the way in which they have developed. The hazard of industrial espionage, suspicion of possible breach of confidence or fear of the activity of antivivisectionists has affected how they have operated. My own experience of membership of more than one LERP has given me evidence of variation in the modus operandi of these ethical committees.

A milestone in the progress of the LERP was the Report of a Workshop on Progressing the Ethical Review Process, convened by Maggy Jennings (RSPCA), Bryan Howard (University of Sheffield) and Graham Moore (Pfizer Central Research) on 22/10/1997. This exercise was further developed as a LASA round table discussion with a Home Office Inspector present as an observer (12/6/1998). The outcome was published by LASA under the title *The Ethical Review Process in Academia*.

The Home Office issued its own document on the LERP in the form of a Supplementary Note by the Chief Inspector in December 2000, supplementary seemingly to Appendix J of the Home Office Guidance. This document appeared on a website as http://www.homeoffice.gov.uk/docs/erp_chief.html on seven pages. This was followed by the issue of the 'Home Office (2001) A(SP)A Inspectorate review of the Ethical Review Process in establishments designated under the A(SP)A, November 2001'. In a letter to certificate holders (22/04/05), the Home Office recommended the RSPCA publication *Resource Book for Lay Members of ERPs*.

In the European arena awareness of an ethical review process was stimulated by the publication of the Final Report of the Sub-Group Ethical Review of the Technical Expert Working Group for the revision of Directive 86/609/EEC on the protection of animals used for experimental purposes. A serious warning accompanied the document: 'The views expressed in this report do not necessarily reflect those of the European Commission but of TEWGER (Technical Expert Working Group on Ethical Review).' Many of the suggestions in the report are already embodied in UK practice, for example:

- local ethical committees (p. 5(iii) – our LERP)
- national committees (p. 5) – our APC with emphasis on the 3Rs)
- Objectives of Ethical Review (p. 3(i)) – our aims of the LERP.

New suggestions were concerned with the keeping of records, to be called an 'audit trail' (p. 10), and the substitution of the 'cost/benefit' expression by 'harm-benefit' (p. 3).

Named animal care and welfare officer (NACWO)

There is an abundance of literature on this topic concerning the named person in day-to-day care – known since January 1997 as the named animal care and welfare officer (NACWO) (PCD Circular 1/97). Particularly useful for study is the IAT booklet *Guidance notes on the role of the named animal care and welfare officer in establishments designated under the Animals (Scientific Procedures) Act 1986.* In a similar fashion the Royal College of Veterinary Surgeons has published material on the role of the named veterinary surgeon in the form of a guide and code of practice (2005). The material published by these two institutions is of practical relevance to their specific roles.

The NACWO, the NVS and the law

The A(SP)A deals with the roles of the NACWO and the NVS in ss. 6 and 7. The subsections involving the roles are (5), (6) and (7). Section 6 is concerned with scientific procedure establishments and s. 7 with breeding and supplying establishments.

'6. (5) A certificate under this section shall specify –
(a) a person to be responsible for the day to day care of the protected animals kept for experimental or other scientific purposes at the establishment; and
(b) a veterinary surgeon or other suitably qualified person to provide advice on their health and welfare;
and the same person may, if the Secretary of State thinks fit, be specified under both paragraphs of this subsection.'

With regard to (5)b, in special circumstances, a non-veterinarian can be appointed to the post, if the Royal College of Veterinary Surgeons approves. This is most common for organisations whose main interest is fish, where veterinary support is not always locally available.

This implies the possibility, but hardly the likelihood in practice, of the NACWO and the NVS being one and the same person.

There is an important variation between subsection 6(6) and subsection 7(6) because of the involvement in scientific procedure establishments of personal licensees:

'6. (6) If it appears to any person specified in a certificate pursuant to subsection (5) above that the health or welfare of any such animal as is mentioned in that subsection gives rise to concern he shall:

(a) notify the person holding a personal licence who is in charge of the animal; or

(b) if there is no such person or it is not practicable to notify him, take steps to ensure that the animal is cared for and, if it is necessary for it to be killed, that it is killed by a method which is appropriate under Schedule 1 to this Act or approved by the Secretary of State.'

'7. (6) If it appears to any person specified in a certificate pursuant to subsection (5) above that the health or welfare of any such animal as is mentioned in that subsection gives rise to concern he shall take steps to ensure that it is cared for and, if it is necessary for it to be killed, that it is killed by a method appropriate under Schedule 1 to this Act or approved by the Secretary of State.'

Subsection (7) is identical in both s. 6 and s. 7;

'In any case to which subsection (6) above applies the person specified in the certificate pursuant to paragraph (a) of subsection (5) above may also notify the person (if different) specified pursuant to paragraph (b) of that subsection; and the person specified pursuant to either paragraph of that subsection may also notify one of the inspectors under this Act.'

In short, if there is concern about an animal the NACWO should notify the personal licensee concerned and may choose to notify the NVS or even an inspector.

Guidance on NACWO

The named animal care and welfare officer will often be a senior animal technician, with an appropriate animal technology qualification, or an experienced stockman with an appropriate qualification in agricultural science. The IAT, understandably, would like this role to be confined to Registered Animal Technicians (RAn.Techs), but there seems little prospect of this occurring in the near future. In most establishments there will be several NACWOs, each responsible for a discrete area of the establishment or an equally discrete area of activity (e.g. production of transgenic mice). Whether the NACWO's role covers an area or an activity, the role should be clearly defined and communication routes established to ensure a standard approach across the establishment. The daily responsibilities, assigned by the Guidance to the NACWO, implies a need to appoint deputies and indeed the mandatory NACWO training, introduced after APC recommendation in 2002, has been extended to cover deputies in most institutions.

Guidance specifies in section 4.57 that it is the NACWO who is expected to ensure the highest standards of husbandry and care, and alludes to ss. 6(6) and 7(6) of the Act with regard to actions taken when an animal's condition gives cause for concern.

Responsibilities of the NACWO

Named Animal Care and Welfare Officers should:

- 'be familiar with the main provisions of the Act;
- have an up-to-date knowledge of laboratory animal technology; be aware of the standards of care, accommodation, husbandry and welfare set out in the relevant Codes of Practice; and take steps to ensure these are met;
- be knowledgeable about relevant methods of humane killing listed in Schedule 1 to the Act (together with any other approved methods listed in the certificate of designation), and either be competent in their use or be able to contact others, named on a register maintained at the establishment, who are;
- know which areas of the establishment are listed in the Schedule to the certificate of designation and the purposes for which their use is approved;
- ensure that every protected animal kept in a designated holding area is seen and checked at least once daily by a competent person;
- know how to contact, at any time, the Named Veterinary Surgeon (or other suitably qualified person) or deputy, and the certificate holder (or nominee). At designated scientific procedure establishments, the NACWO should also know how to contact project and personal licence holders;
- be familiar with the main provisions of the project licences, particularly the adverse effects expected for each protocol, and the control measures and humane endpoints specified;
- assist the certificate holder in ensuring that suitable records are maintained, under the supervision of the veterinary surgeon, of the health of the protected animals; of the environmental conditions in the rooms in which protected animals are held; and of the source and disposal of protected animals; and
- take an active part in the *ethical review process* at the establishment, and advise applicants for licences and licensees on practical opportunities to implement the replacement, reduction and refinement alternatives.'

(Guidance 4.58)

In order for the NACWOs to fulfil these responsibilities, not only must they have an in-depth knowledge of the species housed but they must be able to communicate this to licensees and colleagues, secure in the knowledge that they act with the authority of the certificate holder.

'Certificate holders should ensure that these persons have been clearly entrusted with the necessary management authorities and that their advice on the welfare of animals is sought and taken by project and personal licence holders, of whatever seniority, both at the planning stage and once work is in progress . . .'

(Guidance 4.51)

There is an obligation on prospective project licence holders to seek the advice of the NACWO as regards their proposal project. Refer to the Declarations section, p. 2 of the Project Licence Application.

The delegated authority held by the NACWO should be reinforced by the relationship between the NACWO and the certificate holder; '. . . Direct lines of communication between named persons and the certificate holder should be provided and used effectively' (Guidance 4.49).

The overriding importance of the NACWO both to the institution and the Inspectorate can be gleaned from several sections in the Guidance. As NACWOs have become more science orientated, it has become necessary for institutions to be aware of potential conflicts of interest. As the NACWO is responsible for animal welfare on behalf of the certificate holder, it is deemed inappropriate for a NACWO to fulfil the role of project licence holder for a scientific rather than a service role; in such cases another NACWO should be appointed to oversee the welfare implications of the NACWO's project (Guidance 4.54).

The knowledge base of the NACWO, already extensive, should be constantly upgraded to keep pace with welfare and scientific developments, and it is expected that he or she will be enabled and encouraged to participate in continuing professional development (CPD). This is already expected if the post holder is a RAn.Tech. or a Chartered Biologist.

The other indication of the importance of this post is the requirement for the certificate holder to ensure that the temporary absence or loss of the NACWO does not compromise the welfare or husbandry of the protected animals. Arrangements must be made to cover the NACWO's activities in this eventuality, usually by appointing a deputy, but if the NACWO leaves the post, for whatever reason, they must be replaced quickly by another competent person. Given that the certificate holder must continue to be responsible for the NACWO's performance and either correct any shortcomings or replace the failing individual, it can be seen that this post has become a pivotal one and richly deserves greater remuneration than that of the standard animal care worker.

Named veterinary surgeon (NVS)

The 1998 amendment of the A(SP)A stresses a facet of the role of the NVS as regards animals to be kept alive at the conclusion of a series of procedures. Section 10 states:

'(3D) The conditions of a project licence shall include such conditions as the Secretary of State considers appropriate to ensure: –

(a) that where a protected animal has been subjected to a series of regulated procedures for a particular purpose, at the conclusion of the series a veterinary surgeon or, if none is available, another suitably qualified person determines whether the animal should be killed or kept alive;

(b) that, if that person considers that it is likely to remain in lasting pain or distress, the animal is killed by a method appropriate to the animal under

Schedule 1 to this Act, or by such other method as may be authorised by the personal licence of the person by whom the animal is killed; and

(c) that where the animal is to be kept alive, it is kept at a designated establishment (subject to subsection (6D) below).'

'(6D) The conditions of a certificate issued under section 6 or 7 above [*sic*] shall include such conditions as the Secretary of State considers appropriate to ensure that any animal kept alive after being subjected to a series of regulated procedures will continue to be kept at the establishment under the supervision of a veterinary surgeon or other suitably qualified person unless it is moved to another designated establishment or a veterinary surgeon certifies that it will not suffer if it ceases to be kept at a designated establishment.'

It is to be presumed that the 'veterinary surgeon' in the above text is the NVS of the designated establishment. It could be supposed that 'another qualified person' is the approved non-veterinarian replacement of a NVS, as allowed for in s. 5(b) of the A(SP)A.

A person other than a veterinary surgeon may be accepted in respect of certain species when, after consultation with the Royal College of Veterinary Surgeons, it appears that no appropriate veterinary surgeon is available. In practice, this is unusual and has arisen mostly in relation to establishments in which work is confined to fish or avian embryos.

NVS involved in research

Where the named veterinary surgeon also holds a project licence, a different veterinary surgeon should be nominated to perform the duties of the named veterinary surgeon for the project.

Where the named veterinary surgeon holds only a personal licence, there is no need for a different person to be named as the veterinary surgeon for this work, unless there is a risk of a conflict of interest between the scientific outcome of the research and the welfare of the animals. If such a conflict of interest is thought likely to arise, it will be necessary to obtain the opinion of another veterinary surgeon (who should be identified on the certificate of designation) on matters relating to the health and welfare of the animals involved.

Responsibilities of the NVS

Guidance p. 25:

'The NVS should:

- be familiar with the main provisions of the Act;
- ensure that adequate veterinary cover and services are available at all times, and that the necessary contact details are known to those with relevant responsibilities for the care and welfare of protected animals at the designated establishment;

- visit all parts of the establishment designated in the certificate at a frequency which will allow effective monitoring of the health and welfare of the protected animals under their care;
- notify the personal licensee who is in charge of a protected animal if they become aware that the health or welfare of that animal is giving rise to concern. If there is no such licensee, or if one is not available, the Named Veterinary Surgeon must take steps to ensure that the animal is cared for and, if necessary, that it is humanely killed using an appropriate method. If there is any doubt about what action should be taken, a Home Office inspector should be notified;
- be familiar with relevant methods of humane killing listed in Schedule 1 to the Act, together with any additional approved methods set out in the conditions of the certificate of designation;
- have a thorough knowledge of the husbandry and welfare requirements of the species kept at the establishment (including the prevention, diagnosis and treatment of disease); and be able to advise on quarantine requirements and health screening, and the impact of housing and husbandry systems on the welfare and needs of a protected animal;
- control, supply and direct the use of controlled drugs, prescription-only medicines and other therapeutic substances for use on protected animals in the establishment;
- maintain animal health records to the required professional standard relating to all the protected animals at the establishment, including advice or treatment given; and ensure that such records are readily available to the Named Animal Care & Welfare Officer, the certificate holder and (if requested) the Home Office;
- certify that an animal is fit to travel to a specified place;
- have regular contact with the certificate holder and the Named Animal Care & Welfare Officer(s) and;
- take an active part in the *ethical review process* at the establishment.

At a scientific procedures establishment, the Named Veterinary Surgeon should also:

- advise licensees, applicants and others on how to implement the principles of replacement, reduction and refinement. In particular, to advise about the impact of experimental procedures on the welfare of protected animals; the recognition of pain, suffering, distress or lasting harm; general and experimental surgical techniques, and post-operative care; appropriate methods of general anaesthesia, analgesia and euthanasia; strategies to minimise the severity of protocols, including the recognition or implementation of suitable humane endpoints;
- be familiar with the main provisions of the project licences in use, in particular the adverse effects expected for each protocol; the means by which they are to be avoided, recognised and alleviated; and the humane endpoints to be applied;

- ● ensure that an appropriate clinical investigation or therapy is undertaken
  for the welfare of a protected animal undergoing regulated procedures,
  but that the data or other products being collected as part of the programme of work are not compromised as a result; and
- ● when appropriate, determine that an animal may remain alive at the conclusion of a series of regulated procedures, or certify that its welfare will
  not be compromised if it is removed from the designated place.'

Any relevant forms of certification which may be required will normally be done
by the NVS, in conformity with the guidance of the Royal College of Veterinary
Surgeons on certification and the Twelve Principles of Certification drafted by the
RCVS together with other interested bodies. Updated guidance will be found on
the RCVS website.

Material on the role of the NVS

The Royal College of Veterinary Surgeons in its *RVS Guidance for Named
Veterinary Surgeons employed in Scientific Procedure Establishments and Breeding and Supplying
Establishments under the Animals (Scientific Procedures) Act 1986* (issued November
2004) gives useful information as regards the NVS. For example:

'5) The NVS should: –
- ● provide advice on animal health and welfare to the certificate holder, project and personal licence holders, and animal care staff;
- ● notify the personal licence holder of animals whose condition gives cause
  for concern and, if necessary, arrange for or carry out humane killing if
  this is required;
- ● determine whether an animal remains alive at the end of regulated procedures when this is an option;
- ● certify, as necessary, fitness of animals to leave the establishment;
- ● participate in the establishment's ethical review process; and,
- ● ensure that appropriate records are maintained.'

'11) The names of the veterinary surgeons deputising for the NVS are not
included on the certificate of designation. Therefore, they should be recorded
at the establishment and made known to the certificate holder, the NACWO,
licensees and other relevant staff in the establishment. The means of contact-
ing an appropriate veterinary surgeon at any time should be clearly defined
and available.'

'18) The Home Office requires that a new NVS attend a course, approved
by the RCVS, specifically on the role of the NVS, either before or within
one year of accepting appointment. In any event, a new NVS should undertake training on the needs of the laboratory animals on which he or she will
provide advice.

19) The NVS and veterinary surgeons assisting or deputising for the NVS are expected to participate in continuing professional development relevant to the species held and used and the type of scientific work carried out at the establishment.'

As regards euthanasia, the direct involvement of the NVS with the killing of animals was increased in March 1997 by the new version of Schedule 1. A registered veterinary surgeon may, without a personal licence, kill ungulates by:

(i) destruction of the brain by free bullet; or
(ii) captive bolt, percussion or electrical stunning followed by destruction of the brain or exsanguinations before return of consciousness.

An extra note

The Banner Committee was established to consider the ethical implications of emerging technologies in the breeding of farm animals, and reported in 1995. It was concerned with the welfare of animals involved in such techniques and its comments could be of interest to veterinarians involved in research. Professor Banner was concerned about the adverse effects in genetically modified animals and posited unacceptable 'intrinsically objectionable' modifications which might fall outside the category of 'adverse effects'. The APC Reports 1995 and 1996 (pp. 12–13) commented on the Banner Report which as yet has no direct specific impact on the responsibilities of named persons under the A(SP)A.

Overlapping responsibilities of the NACWO and NVS

The NACWO and NVS are closely associated in both s. 6 and s. 7 of the Act. On both of them is laid the responsibility of dealing with an animal, the health and welfare of which gives rise to concern by subsection (6) of ss. 6 and 7. Both the NACWO and NVS are obliged to notify the relevant personal licence holder, if appropriate, or care for the animal or see that it is killed. Subsection (7) of ss. 6 and 7 of the Act suggests the NACWO might notify the NVS when there is concern about an animal's health and welfare.

It also suggests either the NACWO or the NVS might notify the Inspector in such circumstances.

The very nature of the roles ascribed in law to the NACWO and NVS imply involvement one with the other as well as an amount of overlapping of the duties assigned to either of them. The most onerous duty of the NACWO, the daily checking of every animal, is a prerequisite for the NVS to adequately fulfil his/her main responsibility of monitoring the health and welfare of the animals. The awareness of the NACWO alerts the NVS to attend immediately to the care of specific animals.

The interrelationship between NACWO and NVS requires that:

- The NACWO must ensure health records are maintained in a form determined by the NVS.
- The NACWO must know how to contact the NVS or his/her deputy.
- The duties of the NACWO and NVS as regards euthanasia overlap.
- The NVS must have regular contact with the NACWO.
- The NVS should make the health records available to the NACWO.
- The NVS should make known the identity of nominated deputies to the NACWO.

Background literature on both the NACWO and NVS reinforce the need for these two named persons to be closely associated. The duties of both overlap, particularly in the area of training:

> 'The NACWO may also be given delegated authority for the organisation of training for all animal care personnel . . .'
>
> (NACWO Guidelines, p. 5)

> 'The NVS is in the best position to advise on improvements in anaesthesia, surgical techniques and the control of pain and will be expected to do so. An NVS will also be expected to advise on methods of humane killing and train technicians and scientists in these and other skills.'
>
> (*Guide to Professional Conduct*, 3.7.6)

The NACWO guidelines also state:

> 'The NACWO will be called upon to advise and assist others working under the legislation including . . . the NVS.'
>
> (p. 1)

The *Guide to Professional Conduct* comments:

> 'An NVS must establish a professional working relationship with the Named Persons Responsible for Day-to-Day Care (now the NACWO), who will normally be senior animal technologists with considerable experience in the husbandry of laboratory animals and their use in research, . . .'
>
> (3.7.5)

Figures 9.2 and 9.3 perhaps more clearly illustrate the overlapping and interdependence of the NACWO and NVS.

Home Office correspondence on the role of the NVS

The use of animals for education and training in agriculture

Here follow extracts from Home Office correspondence on various matters germane to the application of the A(SP)A in agriculture and veterinary practice.

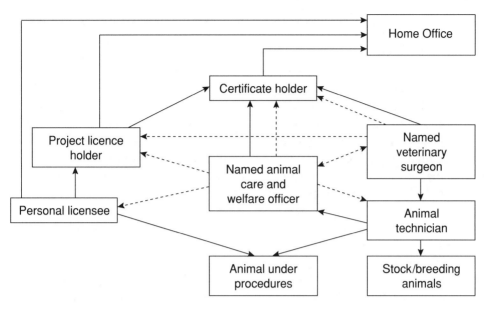

Fig. 9.2 Relationships of named animal care and welfare officer (NACWO) to other members of staff.

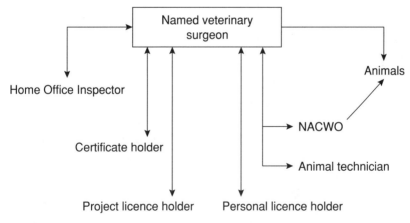

Fig. 9.3 Relationships of named veterinary surgeon (NVS) with other interested parties.

'Section 5(3)(e) of the Animals (Scientific Procedures) Act 1986 permits the application of regulated procedures which may cause pain, suffering, distress or lasting harm to animals for the purpose of education or training otherwise than in primary or secondary schools.

It is Home Office policy to grant project licences authorising regulated procedures only for educational purposes in a scientific context and to restrict the use of animals for training (i.e. the acquisition of manual skills) only to the practice of microsurgery in defined training courses.

This policy precludes the use of animals for demonstrations or practice of techniques in veterinary medicine and agriculture where the aim is to become proficient in performing such techniques. Thus project licences under the Animals (Scientific Procedures) Act cannot be granted for this purpose.

Section 2(8) of the Act has the effect of excluding from control procedures carried out for the purpose of recognised veterinary, agricultural or animal husbandry practice. The use of animals to demonstrate and practise routine techniques such as blood sampling and simple injections for veterinary or agricultural students must comply with legislative controls such as the Veterinary Surgeons Act, the Veterinary Surgeons (Practice by Students) Regulations 1981, and subsequent Statutory Instruments.

In general, this use will need to be restricted to animals which have a perceived need to undergo the sampling or treatment for a specific veterinary or animal husbandry reason. For example, blood samples may be taken for biochemical analysis for diagnosis (or "profiling" with a view to diagnosis) of trace element status and injections may be given if these form part of the routine husbandry of the herd or flock as in vaccination programmes in sheep or iron administration in piglets. The guiding principle in the use of animals in training courses must be that the use must benefit the individual animal or the herd directly.'

(HO, March 1990)

The Animals (Scientific Procedures) Act 1986 and recognised veterinary practice

'The Act provides for the licensing of experimental and other scientific procedures applied to living vertebrate animals which may cause pain, suffering, distress or lasting harm. The controls do not extend to procedures applied to animals in the course of recognised veterinary, agricultural or animal husbandry practice; to procedures for the identification of animals for scientific purposes and which cause no more than momentary pain or distress and no lasting harm; or to clinical tests on animals for evaluating a veterinary product under authority of an Animal Test Certificate (Medicines Act 1968).

In the years since the Act was introduced, the interpretation of "recognised veterinary practice" has caused some difficulties. However, in most cases, the difficulties have been resolved by considering two questions about the proposed action [Fig. 9.4]. Is what you wish to do being performed essentially for a scientific or experimental purpose? If the answer to this is yes, then it is likely that licences under the Animals (Scientific Procedures) Act are required before the work is carried out. The second question should resolve any remaining difficulty; is what you wish to do for the direct benefit of the animal or its immediate group? If the answer to this is yes, then the work could reasonably be considered to be "recognised veterinary practice".

For example, if you wish to take a series of biopsies from an animal for the prime purpose of diagnosis and subsequent monitoring of the effectiveness of

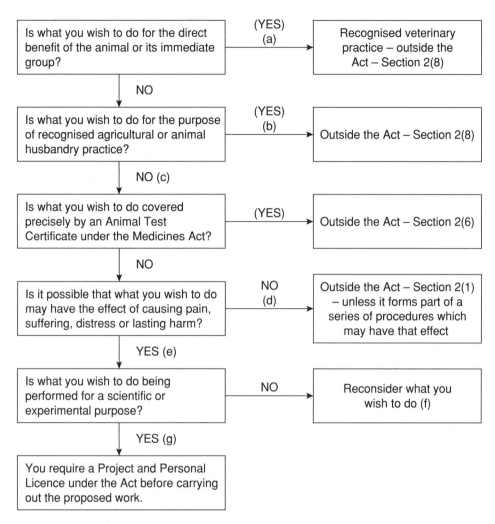

Fig. 9.4 The Animals (Scientific Procedures) Act 1986 and the performance of procedures by veterinary surgeons. Letters in brackets refer to examples of procedures falling within the particular decision and explained in Table 9.2. *Source*: Home Office.

treatment, then this would be "recognised practice". If, however, the biopsies are taken primarily to study the pathogenesis of the condition, then licences would be required as the purpose is now one of scientific enquiry. It is accepted that there will be cases where the difference between these circumstances is less clear but the consideration of the question of benefit to the animal will usually resolve the difficulty.

The status of blood sampling may often be in doubt, particularly in educational and training establishments. Here again, the questions of purpose and benefit will usually provide a clear answer. If the samples are being taken from an animal, or animals within a herd or flock, for the purpose of diagnosis, or for metabolic profile test etc. and, as a result of the analysis of the samples,

Table 9.2 Some terms and examples of their use in practice

Term	Example(s)
(a) direct benefit	taking blood samples from an animal, or animals within a herd, for diagnosis, metabolic profile test, etc. taking a series of biopsies from an animal for diagnosis and monitoring the efficacy of treatment giving veterinary treatment to an experimental animal when treatment is for animal's benefit and not part of the scientific procedure use of drugs in ways other than described in product licence but for direct benefit of animal concerned NB: anaesthesia for a scientific purpose is regulated
(b) recognised practice	embryo transfer testing for halothane susceptibility in pigs restraint in commercial systems laparoscopy for AI laparoscopy for observation of the gonads for sexing birds removal of gonads or hormone administration for control of reproduction in non-experimental situations
(c) not recognised	laparoscopy for observation of the ovaries for a scientific purpose feeding of diets at variance with normal practice restraint in non-commercial or experimental systems
(d) no adverse effect	feeding of diets at variance with normal practice but which are not intended to result in deficiencies or excess of any dietary component and will maintain body weight within 85% of normal growth or starting weight reasonable restraint for short periods, for example a metabolism crate for up to 14 days
(e) adverse effect	any penetration of the integument, i.e. use of needle any procedure requiring sedation or anaesthesia maintenance in close restraint for any period and in restraint for long periods feeding of haematophagous insects
(f) think again	taking into account the provisions of the Veterinary Surgeons Act, the Veterinary Surgeons (Practice by Students) Regulations 1981, the Animal Health Act 1981, the Medicines Act 1968 and the Wildlife and Countryside Act 1981
(g) scientific purposes	taking blood for blood products or laboratory use taking blood for teaching purposes taking biopsies for studying pathogenesis of a condition inoculation of material into an animal for diagnosis of disease in another animal use of substances, drugs, etc. other than as described in product licence, for research/development and not covered by an ATC

action will be taken for the benefit of the animal or animals, then the sampling is clearly "recognised practice". If the samples are intended essentially for laboratory use or for teaching purposes and there is no real prospect of direct benefit to the animal from which the sample was taken, then this would not be considered to be "recognised practice" and would require licences under the Act. The particular case of blood donor animals in clinical practice has been considered by the Preliminary Investigation and Advisory Committee of the Royal College. Their advice is set out in the Guide to Professional Conduct, 1990 Edition, Appendix 12.2.

Special problems in interpretation may arise for veterinary surgeons when dealing with animals undergoing a scientific procedure under the Act. The administration of an anaesthetic agent as part of the procedure described in the project licence or the performance of any other part of the procedure can only be legally carried out if the veterinary surgeon holds a personal licence. However, if the animal undergoing the scientific procedure requires clinical attention from the veterinary surgeon, usually from a cause extraneous to the scientific procedure itself, then no licence is necessary for carrying out the clinical procedure on the animal.

In any case of difficulty where you are unable to reach a decision in this matter, you should seek advice from the Home Office Inspectorate. The addresses of the Regional Offices are shown in Appendix 10 of the RCVS Register and Directory.'

(Jeremy Roberts, HO Inspector, 10 October 1990)

Further guidance

The list of examples in Table 9.2 is illustrative and not exhaustive. The advice of the Home Office Inspector should always be sought in cases of doubt.

An informative document on *The Veterinary Surgeons Act 1966 and the Animals (Scientific Procedures) Act 1986 – acts of veterinary surgery performed by non-veterinarians* was issued by the Royal College of Veterinary Surgeons on 7 September 1998. It was accompanied by an LAVA Position Paper on *The Veterinary Surgeons Act 1966 and the Animals (Scientific Procedures) Act 1986 – a conflict of legislative requirements.* Both these documents, available from the Royal College or LAVA, could be of interest to the NVS. Another worthwhile publication of the Royal College of Veterinary Surgeons is *Legislation Affecting the Veterinary Profession in the UK* (6th edn).

Chapter 10

Codes of Practice

As a response to the introduction of the A(SP)A, the Royal Society and the Universities Federation for Animal Welfare, after wide consultation, issued detailed guidelines for the housing and care of animals in scientific procedures. The government accepted these guidelines and made them the basis of the Code of Practice.

There are currently four codes of practice in operation which were issued under s. 21 of the A(SP)A.

- Housing and Care of Animals used in Scientific Procedures (1989)
- Housing and Care of Animals in Designated Breeding and Supplying Establishments (1995)
- Humane Killing of Animals under Schedule 1 to the Animals (Scientific Procedures) Act 1986 (1997) (cf. Chapter 5)
- Housing and Care of Pigs Intended for use as Xenotransplant Source Animals (1999)

An erstwhile code of practice on Licensing and Inspection under the A(SP)A, issued in 1994, was replaced by a Charter on Licensing and Inspection in 2000. A document akin to a code of practice, *Results of a Survey of Dog Accommodation and Care*, was issued in 1999. It has a similar construct to the existing codes and is given similar status on the Home Office website.

The codes of practice concerned with the operation of the Inspectorate and with euthanasia are referred to in Chapters 14 and 20. The two welfare codes – (a) for the Housing and Care of Animals used in Scientific Procedures; and (b) for the Housing and Care of Animals in Designated and Supplying Establishments (supplemented in 1999 for Ferrets and Gerbils) – have as their scope the basis of good husbandry to ensure suitable standards of animal welfare. These codes are the legal expression of Article 5 of the European Convention for the Protection of Vertebrate Animals used for Experimental and other Scientific Procedures. This expression has become reality recently as the result of a large-scale European-wide consultation exercise culminating in the Draft Appendix A to ETS No. 123. That this highly detailed document covering virtually all types of experimental animal will come into force from 15 June 2007.

Currently the Convention states:

'Any animal used or intended for use in a procedure shall be provided with accommodation, an environment, at least a minimum degree of freedom of movement, food, water, care appropriate to its health and well being. Any restriction on the extent to which an animal can satisfy its physiological and ethological needs shall be limited as far as practicable.'

There is little purpose to be served by reproducing the various texts in this chapter since the position of the codes will always be fluid, developing in the light of new published and practical knowledge, but the reader should bear in mind that a code of practice represents the minimum standard to be obtained within an establishment and practitioners will be encouraged by Inspectors to develop their units to meet evolving standards as recognised by their peers, thus promoting best practice.

Present welfare codes

The current codes can be viewed and downloaded from the Home Office website and every unit within an establishment should have access to a printed copy. All active practitioners should be fully conversant with the material in these codes. It is not expected that individuals commit to memory all the fine detail of cage sizes relevant to the animal's weight and the exact environmental ranges that should pertain; however, it is expected that those people with a role under the A(SP)A, especially the NACWO, should have access to this information and know how to implement it with regard to good husbandry and welfare.

Code of Practice for the Housing and Care of Animals used in Scientific Procedures (COPHCASP)

The topics which define the scope of this code include:

- the animal house, its facilities, its staff and their safety and security
- the environment provided for the animals within the unit
- the sources, care and health of the animals
- transport, feeding, watering, handling and cleaning
- husbandry needs of certain species
- the health status of the animals
- tables of environmental data and cage sizes for the housing of growing animals.

The Home Office Inspectorate has carried out audits of both commercial (1993) and academic (1996) establishments (APC Report 1997 p. 14) to ensure compliance with the Code of Practice.

Code of Practice for the Housing and Care of Animals in Designated Breeding and Supplying Establishments

This Code consists of two parts. The first part deals with the welfare in general pertinent to species listed in Schedule 2 of the A(SP)A. The second part deals separately in more detail with each of the species involved. It is supplemented with a draft code specifically for ferrets and gerbils (1999). The information in these codes is now found on the Home Office website with 27 publications grouped under the heading 'Codes of Practice and Guidance Notes', which allows the practitioner to download the codes for the species specifically of interest.

In a fresh approach, the Home Office has included in this section 'Guidance Notes' and 'Supplementary Guidance' which cover such topics as 'Projects that Generate and/or Maintain Genetically Modified Animals'; 'The Ethical Review Process'; 'The Conduct of Regulatory Toxicology and Safety Evaluation Studies'; 'Projects for Educational Purposes'; 'Breeding Supply of Laboratory Animals in the UK'; 'Non-rodent Selection in Pharmacological Toxicology'. Those items classified as guidance appear to be aimed at Project Licence Holders and 'Named Persons' especially, although they would also be of interest to personal licensees.

The Charter

Large parts of the Charter on Licensing and Inspection are the same as the original Code of Practice for Licensing and Inspection but it probably lacks the full legal force of a full-blown code of practice. Key points of the Charter are:

- target time to issue a licence from receipt of inspector's recommendation increased from 10 to 15 days
- no targets set for the time inspectors need to consider applications
- 'paramount' need to minimise animal use and suffering and to maximise the standard of care
- confirmation that inspectors will be available to discuss and help refine proposals ahead of submission of applications.

(Cf. *Research Defence Society News*, January 2000, p. 4)

Dog Care

A consequence of the Channel 4 *Countryside Undercover* programme 'It's a Dog's Life' (March 1997) was the recommendations resulting from the survey of dog accommodation referred to above.

- Dogs should be housed in groups or pairs, unless persuasive veterinary, husbandry or scientific reasons can be provided for single housing. Socialisation programmes should be adopted for dogs held singly/in small groups.
- Pens should be cleaned daily, with waste material being replaced with fresh bedding. Pen design must offer some environmental complexity and choice.
- Where restraint/confinement is required, justification must be included in the project licence application with details of measures to provide high welfare standards.

- Staff training should completely cover welfare including housing, husbandry, handling, behaviour and health.
- Environmental enrichment and welfare as well as training and assessment of competency should be considered in the LERP.

   (*Research Defence Society News*, January 1999 and APC Report 1998, p. 19)

Legal force of the codes

The legal basis for these codes of practice is s. 21 of the A(SP)A where the Secretary of State is encouraged to use his enabling powers to produce subordinate legislation in the form of codes of practice.

'21. (2) The Secretary of State shall issue codes of practice as to the care of protected animals and their use for regulated procedures and may approve such codes issued by other persons.'

Subsection (3) provides for consultation with the APC in respect of these codes. Subsections (5) and (6) give the details of the parliamentary process for bringing the codes into law.

It is only subsection (4) that has practical significance for those involved with protected animals in research:

'21. (4) A failure on the part of any person to comply with any provision of a code issued or approved under subsection (2) above shall not of itself render that person liable to criminal or civil proceedings but: –

(a)   any such code shall be admissible in evidence in any such proceedings; and

(b)   if any of its provisions appears to the court conducting the proceedings to be relevant to any question arising in the proceedings it shall be taken into account in determining that question.'

In short, one cannot be prosecuted for breaching a stipulation of any of the codes. If, however, one were to be accused of an offence – for example, causing an animal unnecessary suffering – then any relevant provision of the codes would be considered. If any such provision had been flouted the burden of proof, usually borne solely by the prosecution, would roll over partly on to the accused. He/she would now have to establish that the method of care he/she used was as good as, if not better than, the method of care proposed by the code. This would be a difficult proposition to establish to the satisfaction of any court. In practice, however, the codes are used to establish minimum standards of care which in most cases would be exceeded by scientific institutions. They set out, as a rule, to outline standards of facilities and care regimes which are regarded as 'fit for purpose', and taken as a whole with the supplementary guidance notes issued from time to time, provide a basis if not necessarily for best practice, which is constantly being refined, then certainly for acceptable practice within scientific discipline.

One should always remember that codes and guidance are not meant to represent a status quo within a biological facility but that new innovations, provided they are ethically justified, should be introduced as and when an institution feels able to do so.

Chapter 11

The Re-use of Animals

This much-debated topic, at least at 5th module sessions for applicants for project licences, has an interesting legal history. The introduction of modifying terms such as 'continued use' or even 'repeated use' did not contribute to clarification of the situation. Section 14 of A(SP)A which deals with the restriction on re-use of animals was effected by the 1998 amendment of the Act. An absolute prohibition was introduced regarding re-use of any animal that would involve severe pain or distress, or any further use of an animal if that animal had already suffered severe pain or distress in a previous regulated procedure (cf. Guidance, n. 5.64). The Guidance has clarified the topic by clear definition of the term 'use' in this context. It also explains the observation of the amended section in practice.

The endemic theoretical confusion may be obviated by adherence to the specific advice given by the inspector involved.

- *Use* – 'The "use" of a protected animal on a protocol extends from the time the animal is issued from stock and the protocol begins, until the observations or the collection of data (or other product) are complete or the animal is killed.' (n. 5.55)

  'Where there is a need to obtain blood samples from an animal that has received a specific pre-treatment, the use of the animal encompasses both the dosing and sampling. Similarly, in the case of a protocol for polyclonal antibody production, use on a single protocol spans the pre-immunisation bleed, the immunisation (and re-immunising) and the blood harvesting.'

  (n. 5.56)

- *Continued use* – This must be specifically authorised by the Secretary of State.

  'If, after a protocol authorized by a project licence has been completed, the animal is being used in a second or subsequent protocol as a matter of scientific necessity, and a naïve animal would not suffice, then this constitutes "continued use".'

  (n. 5.59)

  'A common example is the production of genetically or surgically prepared animals on one protocol and their subsequent use in separate protocols requiring animals of that description.

Similarly, the transfer of protected animals from a protocol on an expiring project licence to its equivalent on a new project licence provided continuity of authority is also considered to be "continued use".'

(n. 5.58)

- *Re-use* – All re-use must be specifically authorised by the Secretary of State. If after a series of regulated procedures for a specific purpose authorised by a project licence has been completed an animal is used in a second or subsequent protocol, and a naïve animal would have sufficed, then there has been 're-use' of this animal within the terms of s. 14 of A(SP)A. Repeated samples of normal blood taken from an animal to prepare blood products, when each sample could equally well have come from a naïve animal, constitutes 're-use'.

The Secretary of State can only authorise the 're-use' of animals which have been subjected to a series of regulated procedures for a particular purpose under a general anaesthetic if

(1) the procedure for which the general anaesthetic was given consisted only of surgical preparation essential for the subsequent procedure (for example, the preparation of animals with carotid artery loops);

(2) the general anaesthetic was administered solely to immobilise the animal and not to prevent pain;

(3) if the 're-use' will be under general anaesthetic and the animal will not be allowed to recover consciousness.

Chapter 12

Records, Returns and Reports

Records

These essential features of the observance in practice of the A(SP)A are usually only the immediate concern of the individual directly involved. It seems appropriate to deal with the matter in categories associated with persons with defined responsibilities under the Act. Specific legal demands, for example s. 10(6)(b), are presented in more detail in the Guidance which is used as the source of the following material. It is the obligation of the persons listed below to provide the requisite records or at least to ensure the provision of them by someone under their authority; for example, an NACWO may be responsible, on a day-to-day basis, for records associated with the CH.

The certificate holder

- Daily records of environmental conditions in enclosed animal holding areas.
- Details of all project and personal licences at the establishment. The records should cover at least the current and the preceding fee period.
- Records of all protected animals bred or obtained for use, supplied for use, or used in regulated procedures. These records should account for each protected animal, except in the case of immature forms (foetal, larval or embryonic stages) which may be recorded in batches until they are issued for use in regulated procedures. The details required, if appropriate, are in the case of:
  (1) *Animals* – species and breed or strain, the type of harmful mutant, genetic modification or surgical modification; approximate age on arrival; sex; if female, whether pregnant; identification number or code (by individual or group number, as appropriate); microbiological status (for example, gnotobiotic) and dates in and out of quarantine or isolation.
  (2) *Source* – the name and address of the breeder or supplier of Schedule 2 animals; the name and address, and number of the authorising project licence, of the UK source of any harmful mutant, genetically modified animal or surgically prepared animal; date of arrival of the animal (or date of birth at that breeding establishment); and date of transfer to holding unit or user unit.

(3) *Use* – the numbers and types of animals allocated as breeding stock; held for supply or use; and at a user establishment, the project licence to which the animal was issued.

(4) *Disposal* (other than to a project licence) – killed by an appropriate method listed in Schedule 1 (or other method authorised in the certificate of designation) whether on welfare grounds, for harvesting tissues for experimental or other scientific purposes, or as surplus to requirements; deaths from other causes; supplied to another designated establishment; discharged from the controls of the Act (for example, to a farm, as a pet, back to stock, to a slaughterhouse, to the wild or supplied for export).

These records should be kept for at least five years after the death or release of the animal, whichever is the longer. They are not intended to be merely preserved but should be used within the establishment to monitor and improve animal welfare. They must be available to the inspector on request who may require further relevant material if need be (cf. Guidance, nn. 4.27–33).

The project licence holder

Provision of full, accurate, contemporary records of regulated procedures is a responsibility of the project licence holder.

'The records should include the following information:
- the project number, the name of the project licence holder and where applicable the names of the deputy project licence holders;
- the name of the personal licensees performing regulated procedures authorised by the project licence;
- details of the regulated procedures and protocols applied, including the type and species of protected animals used;
- a running tally of the numbers of each species used in each protocol;
- the sex and approximate age of the animals at the commencement of the protocols;
- the identification numbers of the animals used (where appropriate);
- the date of commencement of protocols;
- a brief description of the procedures applied;
- the morbidity or mortality produced;
- the date on which protocols were concluded;
- the fate of animals at the end of the regulated procedures (for example, killed within the establishment, released to the wild, released to private care, or released for slaughter);
- details of any continued use or re-use;
- copies of any veterinary (or other) certification and advice received.'

(Guidance, nn. 5.67–8)

Personal licence holder

Adequate records of all regulated procedures performed and whether they were supervised should be kept, together with details of any resulting morbidity or mortality (cf. Guidance, n. 6.19).

Named veterinary surgeon

Animal health records relating to all the protected animals in the establishment should be kept with records of the advice and training given (cf. Guidance, n. 4.62).

Named animal care and welfare officer

Assists the CH by maintaining suitable records, under the supervision of the NVS, of the health of the protected animals; of the environmental conditions in the rooms in which protected animals are held; and of the source and disposal of protected animals. (cf. Guidance, n. 4.58.)

Identification of animals

This legal obligation, the ultimate responsibility of the CH, in practice is laid upon the personal licence holder. The personal licence holder must ensure that all cages, pens or other enclosures are labelled so that those with responsibility under the Act can identify the relevant project licence number, the protocol (the project licence 19b number or short title), the date the protocol was started and the responsible personal licensee. A code may be used as long as it would be possible for the inspector to decode the information. (cf. Guidance, n. 6.20.)

The CH must ensure that cages or confinement areas containing protected animals not undergoing regulated procedures carry a label with a cage/area reference and an identification of the animals held (by individual or batch as appropriate).

The 1998 amendment of A(SP)A paid special attention to the identification of dogs, cats, primates, equidae and other farm animals and adult birds. The identification of each animal is stipulated and stringent regulations are laid down concerning dogs, cats and primates. Those involved in these specialised fields will be fully aware of what is required. The details can be found in the Guidance at n. 4.26.

Returns

'Condition 10 on every project licence:
The project licence holder shall send to the Secretary of State, before the 31 January each year (and within 28 days of the licence having expired or been revoked), a report in a form specified by the Secretary of State, giving

details of the number of procedures and animals used, and the nature and purpose of the procedures performed under the authority of the project licence during the calendar year.'

This is not the place to produce the form issued for returns. All interested parties will receive copies accompanied by full instructions on how to complete the form. Another reason for not producing details in this context is that the requirements for the relevant information have tended to vary. There was a revision of the form in 1990. This was to conform with instructions from the European Commission. Appropriate adjustments were also made to better assess the occurrence of re-use.

Some of the bewilderment associated with the Return may be alleviated if we realise that the questions are intended to produce a comprehensive picture of:

- the species of animals used
- the number of animals used
- the stage of development of the animals used
- the genetic status of the animals used
- the anaesthetics or neuromuscular blocking agents (if any) used
- the reason for animal use
- the nature of the procedures
- the number of procedures
- re-use.

It is important to realise that this exercise is for statistical purposes. It is not another assessment of the project; it is not a demand for a description of the project so far. It is a request to answer specific questions about the use of animals.

It is worth mentioning, as always, that consultation with your inspector would prove helpful should you encounter difficulties in filling in the return.

The aim of the exercise is to gather valid data for the annual publication of *Statistics of Scientific Procedures on Living Animals*. Eventually this information may be merged into a European Report.

The following statistics (Figs. 12.1 to 12.4), available on the Home Office Science and Research website, are samples of the material extracted from the annual returns, published in *Statistics of Scientific Procedures on Living Animals in Great Britain in 2004*, London, HMSO (Cm.6713), 2005.

The figures illustrate the extent and nature of animal experimentation in the UK, but only in 2004 – frozen in time, as it were. These figures, however, do not vary overmuch from one year to the next. Figures from the past indicate the trends of animal use under the A(SP)A.

The total number of scientific procedures started in 2004 was just over 2.85 million, a rise of about 63,000 (2.3%) on 2003 (2.79 million); 85% of the animals used were rodents, while fish made up 7% and birds 4%. Dogs, cats, horses and non-human primates, afforded special protection under the A(SP)A, were used in less than 1% of the procedures. Genetically modified animals were used in 32% of all procedures; 96% of them were rodents.

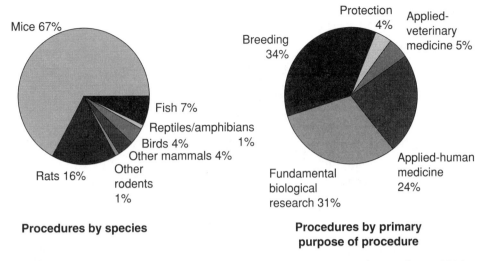

Procedures by species

Procedures by primary purpose of procedure

Fig. 12.1   Procedures by species of animal and primary purpose of procedures, 2004 (cm.6713 p. 14).

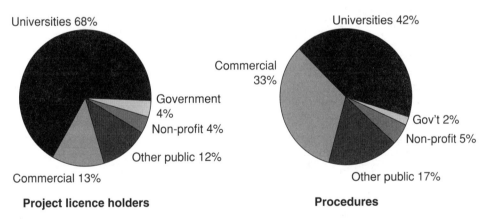

Project licence holders

Procedures

Fig. 12.2   Project licence holders and procedures started in 2004, by type of designated place (cm.6713 p. 21). Note: only those project licence holders reporting procedures in 2004 are included.

Useful statistics were also published in the Animals (Scientific Procedures) Inspectorate *Annual Report 2004.* Although only for one specific year, these figures reflect the average annual workload of the Inspectorate.

In 2004 (July) there were:

- 2,924 project licences in operation (p. 10)
- 573 project licence applications recommended (p. 10)
- 1,645 amendments assessed (p. 10)
- 13,836 personal licences in operation (p. 13)

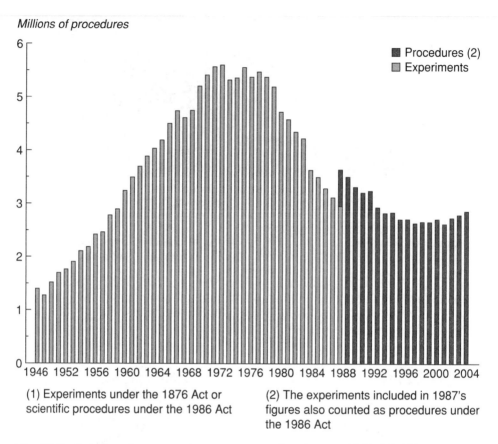

(1) Experiments under the 1876 Act or scientific procedures under the 1986 Act

(2) The experiments included in 1987's figures also counted as procedures under the 1986 Act

Fig. 12.3 Experiments or procedures commenced each year, 1946–2004.[1]

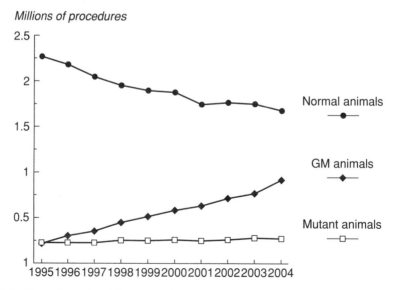

Fig. 12.4 Procedures involving normal, mutant and genetically modified animals, 1995–2004.

Table 12.1 Licence applications and amendments over the five-year period 2000 to 2004

Year	Licence applications assessed	Amendment proposals assessed	Totals
2000	3282	6499	9781
2001	2918	6016	8934
2002	3294	6351	9645
2003	3231	5979	9210
2004	2823	5963	8786

Animals (Scientific Procedures) Inspectorate Annual Report (p. 12).

- 2,248 personal licence applications assessed (p. 9)
- 3,945 personal licence amendments and reviews assessed (p. 9)
- 226 designated establishments (p. 13)
- 2 certificates of designation granted (p. 9)
- 373 amendments requested for certificates of designation (p. 9)

Table 12.1 indicates the number of licence applications and amendments over the five-year period 2000 to 2004.

Reports

Condition 12 on the project licence states:

> 'The project licence holder shall submit such other reports as the Secretary of State may from time to time require.'

Condition 11 deals with a similar theme:

> 'The project licence holder shall maintain a list of publications resulting from the licensed programme of work and a copy of any such publication shall be made available to the Secretary of State on request. The list shall, on request, be submitted to the Secretary of State or made available to be seen by an Inspector, and it shall be submitted to the Secretary of State when the licence is returned to him on expiry or for revocation.'

A significant feature of both these conditions is the contingent terms in which they are couched. They come into operation only either on request or in stipulated circumstances.

Chapter 13

Offences, Penalties, Prosecutions and Peripheral Litigation

A quote from *Hansard* indicates a certain lack of clarity in official information on this topic.

> '**Mr. Baker**: To ask the Secretary of State for the Home Department how many prosecutions have been initiated in respect of cruelty inflicted on animals in the course of approved experiments for each year since 1980; and if he will make a statement. [33017]
>
> **Mr. George Howarth** [*holding answer 6 March 1998*]: Prosecutions for such an offence would be instigated under the Protection of Animals Act 1911 Offences of Cruelty to Animals. The Court Proceeding database, held centrally, can identify only the number of prosecutions brought under the act irrespective of circumstances. However, further sources of information [*11 March 1998: Column: 203*] suggest that there had been no prosecutions, in England and Wales, for cruelty to animals during the course of approved experiments.'

Another quote from an official source confirms the possibility of confusion concerning the application of the A(SP)A in practice.

> 'Our last Circular (on 14 December) reported a *Sunday Times* story which had just been published. There was no truth in the claim that the Home Secretary had banned the use of dogs in scientific procedures and a prompt press agency statement scotched further mis-reporting.
>   Unfortunately, Elliot Morley (Minister at MAFF) compounded the matter by confirming – in an adjournment debate called on 14 December – that dogs would no longer be used. At our Minister's suggestion, Mr Morley has written to those speaking in the Parliamentary debate to retract his statement.'
> (HO PCD Circular 1/100, 22/02/2000)

In light of the above, I will adhere closely to authoritative sources on the subject.

Offences

The Report of the Animal Procedures Committee for 1991 presents in a clear manner salient offences against the 1986 Act. The report precedes its outlining of these offences by a reference to the most important piece of legislation which protects animals:

'9.2 The Act not only controls the way in which scientific procedures on living animals are regulated, but also provides some exemption from the Protection of Animals Act 1911 (1912 in Scotland) for licence holders who are performing authorised procedures under the 1986 Act. However, where unauthorised procedures are being conducted, this immunity is not conferred and it would be possible to bring charges under the 1911 or 1912 Acts.'

The report then indicates offences specific to the 1986 Act:

'9.3 The main criminal offences in the Act relating to the performance of animal procedures can be set out broadly as follows:
   (i)   An offence is committed by anybody who carries out a regulated procedure on a protected animal if:
      (a)   he does not hold a personal licence authorising him to carry out that procedure on that animal;
      (b)   the procedure or species of animal used is not authorised by a project licence; and
      (c)   the procedure is carried out somewhere other than a place authorised both in the personal licence and in the project licence (this is normally an establishment covered by a certificate of designation).
   The person who carries out the procedure is not guilty of the offence of acting without the authority of a project licence if he can show that he reasonably believed, after making due enquiry, that he had proper authority.
   (ii)   An offence is committed by any project licence holder who procures or knowingly permits anybody under his control to carry out a regulated procedure either not authorised by the project licence or outside the authority of that person's personal licence.
   (iii)   No offence under paragraph (i) above is committed by a personal licensee's assistant if the assistant carries out, under the personal licensee's direction and if they are authorised by the personal licence, subordinate duties permitted by the Home Secretary, examples of which are listed in Guidance 6.22–6.27. The personal licence must contain specific authorisation for the use of assistants. A personal licensee cannot delegate the authority of his licence to anybody else, but anybody who carries out a procedure which somebody else, but not he, is allowed to do by a personal licence, commits the offence described in paragraph (i) above.
   (iv)   It is an offence to re-use an animal if the animal has previously been used in a series or combination of procedures carried out for a different purpose and one or more of those procedures consisted of

giving the animal a general anaesthetic. The exceptions to this general rule are if the animal is under a general anaesthetic throughout the further procedures and is not allowed to recover consciousness; or if the anaesthetic was given only for surgical preparation, or only to immobilise the animal. But in any such case, the re-use must have been authorised in advance. It is also an offence, except where specifically authorised, to re-use an animal if the animal has previously been used in a series of procedures for a different purpose, even when none of those procedures involved giving the animal a general anaesthetic.

(v)   The Act requires that an animal which has been used in a series of procedures carried out for any one purpose, and which at the conclusion of the series is suffering or is likely to suffer adverse effects, must immediately be killed or caused to be killed by the personal licensee, either by a Schedule 1 method of humane killing, or by some other method authorised in the personal licence of the person who carries out the killing. A personal licensee who does not comply with this requirement commits an offence.

(vi)   It is an offence to use a neuromuscular blocking agent unless expressly authorised to do so by the personal and project licences under which the procedure is carried out, or to use a neuromuscular blocking agent instead of an anaesthetic. Should a neuromuscular blocking agent be used without authority the person who carried out the procedure is not guilty of the offence if he shows that he reasonably believed, after making due enquiry, that he had that authority.

(vii)   If an Inspector considers that a protected animal is undergoing excessive suffering, it is an offence to fail to comply with the Inspector's requirement that the animal must immediately be killed either by a Schedule 1 method of humane killing or by another method authorised in the personal licence held by a personal licensee.

(viii)   In addition, breaches of standard licence conditions 1 to 5 of a project licence and standard conditions 1 to 10 of a personal licence may also constitute criminal offences.'

The Act also prohibits wrongful disclosure of information.

'1)   Disclosure of information obtained in the exercise of functions under the Act otherwise than for the purpose of discharging those functions, providing there are reasonable grounds for believing that the information was given in confidence. This prohibition is not intended to interfere with the performance of proper duties under the Act, such as an inspector consulting another inspector about an application for a licence (s. 24).

2)   Running a breeding or supplying establishment for experimental animals without the necessary designation (s. 22(3)(a) and refer to s. 7(1) and (2)).

3) Presenting a regulated procedure as an exhibition to the general public or for live showing on television for reception by the general public or advertising such a performance to the general public. It is not an offence to allow otherwise authorised procedures to be included in pre-recorded programmes. Nor is it an offence to allow bona fide visitors to laboratories to witness the performance of procedures (s. 22(3)(a) and refer to s. 16).

4) Giving, knowingly and recklessly, information known to be false for the purpose of obtaining or assisting another person to obtain a licence or certificate under the Act (s. 23).

5) Obstructing intentionally a constable or inspector if the constable has been granted a search warrant, or refusing on demand to give the constable or inspector his name and address or gives a false name and address (s. 25(3)(a) and (b)).'

Penalties under the A(SP)A

The Act itself is quite specific in the matter of penalties. The topic is fully dealt with in ss. 22, 23, 24 and 25. A penalty not exceeding two years' imprisonment or a fine or both on conviction on indictment, or not exceeding six months' imprisonment or a fine not exceeding the statutory maximum or both on summary conviction, may be incurred for:

- performing or being involved in unauthorised regulated procedures (refer s. 3)
- contravening s. 1 (causing unnecessary suffering) of the Protection of Animals Act 1911 in a designated establishment (refer s. 22(5))
- breach of confidentiality (refer s. 24).

A penalty, on summary conviction, not exceeding three months' imprisonment or a fine not exceeding the fourth level on the standard scale or both may be incurred for:

- breach of Schedule 2 (refer s. 7);
- re-use without the appropriate consent (refer s. 14);
- not providing authorised euthanasia at the conclusion of regulated procedures when an animal may suffer (refer s. 15);
- performing exhibitions of regulated procedures or advertising the same (refer s. 16);
- use of neuromuscular blocking agent without observing the relevant conditions (refer s. 17);
- refusing to comply with an Inspector's order concerning euthanasia (refer s. 18(3));
- making false or misleading statements in order to obtain a licence or certificate (refer s. 23);
- obstructing or misleading a constable or Inspector acting under s. 25(3).

Prosecution under the Act

The process of prosecution for offences under the Act is set out in s. 26:

'(1) No proceedings for –
   (a) an offence under this Act; or
   (b) an offence under section 1 of the Protection of Animals Act 1911 which is alleged to have been committed in respect of an animal at a designated establishment,
   shall be brought in England and Wales except by or with the consent of the Director of Public Prosecutions.

(2) Summary proceedings for an offence under this Act may (without prejudice to any jurisdiction exercisable apart from this subsection) be taken against any person at any place at which he is for the time being.

(3) Notwithstanding anything in section 127(1) of the Magistrates' Courts Act 1980, any information relating to an offence under this Act which is triable by a magistrates' court in England and Wales may be so tried if it is laid at any time within three years after the commission of the offence and within six months after the date on which evidence sufficient in the opinion of the Director of Public Prosecutions to justify the proceedings comes to his knowledge.

(4) Notwithstanding anything in section 331 of the Criminal Procedure (Scotland) Act 1975, summary proceedings for an offence under this Act may be commenced in Scotland at any time within three years after the commission of the offence and within six months after the date on which evidence sufficient in the opinion of the Lord Advocate to justify the proceedings comes to his knowledge; and subsection (3) of that section shall apply for the purposes of this subsection as it applies for the purposes of that section.

(5) For the purposes of subsections (3) and (4) above a certificate of the Director of Public Prosecutions or, as the case may be, the Lord Advocate as to the date on which such evidence as is there mentioned came to his knowledge shall be conclusive evidence of that fact.'

In s. 29(7) it is pointed out that the words 'Northern Ireland' should, where appropriate be substituted for 'England and Wales'.

Prosecutions in practice

The APC in its 1991 Report (pp. 12–13) took the opportunity not only to highlight and comment on the first prosecution under the A(SP)A but also to reflect on a near-prosecution and on a possible breach of the Act:

'3.8 1991 saw the first successful prosecution under the Act. During the course of a routine inspection of a user establishment, it came to light that a commercial rabbit breeding company, which was not designated under section 7 of the Act to supply animals for scientific use, had supplied rabbits for such use. The user establishment had been led to believe that the company was properly designated and indeed had itself drawn the matter to the attention of the Inspector. As the breeding and supplying company was not designated under the Animals (Scientific Procedures) Act 1986, the Home Office had no powers to investigate the matter itself. It therefore reported the matter to the police, who carried out an investigation and referred it for prosecution. The breeding and supplying company was subsequently convicted under the Act of breeding and supplying animals for use in scientific procedures while not being designated under section 7 of the Act.

Referral for possible prosecution under the Act

3.9 The Committee was most disturbed to learn the details of a very serious case involving a series of infringements in an institution. The infringements involved the application of unauthorised surgical procedures to pigs, including instances of unauthorised re-use, some of which could not have been authorised under the terms of the Act even if authority had been applied for. It was also clear that there had been a lack of post-operative care which had undoubtedly caused avoidable animal suffering. The Home Office referred the matter to the prosecuting authorities in view of the serious nature of the infringements revealed.

3.10 We fully supported this action in referring to the prosecuting authorities what was clearly a very serious series of infringements. While we recognise that decisions on whether or not to prosecute are properly the responsibility of the prosecuting authorities, it was a matter of considerable disappointment that, in the event, the prosecuting authorities decided not to bring charges against those involved. We made our concern known to the Home Office who were later able, with the agreement of the prosecuting authorities, to set out for the Committee the considerations which led to the decision. It was clear that there were highly unusual evidential problems peculiar to this case which would have materially reduced the likelihood of a successful prosecution. We are keen to ensure that any general lessons from this case are learnt for the future and the Home Office has discussed these matters with the prosecuting authorities. It is our view that the failure to prosecute in this case does not reveal any deficiencies in the provisions of the Act itself.

3.11 Although criminal charges were not brought against the project licence holder and the personal licensee involved, it was still open to the Home Office subsequently to take administrative action. Having considered the details of the case, the Home Secretary decided to seek the revocation of all the project licences and the personal licence of the project licence holder, and the personal licence of the personal licensee. We fully support this tough administrative action. Discussions are continuing with the institution where the infringements took place to ensure that it has in place proper controls to avoid a recurrence.'

The possible breach considered in depth by the APC could prove of special interest to 'old timers'.

'3.12 In our last report, we referred to the case of Professor W S Feldberg and Mr J P Stean who had conducted procedures on apparently under-anaesthetised animals. The Committee considered the general lessons to be learnt from this case which led to the recommendations in paragraphs 2.28 and 2.33 of that report about the need to ensure the proper control of licence holders who are passed retirement age.

3.13 In considering the general lessons of this case, we took note of the report of the inquiry by a team led by Sir Brian Bailey established by the Medical Research Council. One outstanding matter from Sir Brian Bailey's report was the allegation that offences under the Act had been committed in that regulated procedures had been conducted before the appropriate project licence authority had been granted. Having considered the evidence available to the inquiry team the Government decided not to refer the case to the prosecuting authorities. In answer to a Parliamentary Question from Sir John Wheeler JP MP (Westminster North), the Rt Hon Mrs Angela Rumbold MP CBE said:

"... We have now completed consideration of the evidence of possible breaches of the 1986 Act, including Professor Feldberg's notebooks, which the MRC forwarded to the Home Office.

We do not consider that, in all the circumstances of the case, there are grounds to justify referring the matter to the Director of Public Prosecutions. As soon as it was clear that avoidable suffering had been caused to animals, the Home Office took action to remove the personal and project licences held by Professor Feldberg and Mr Stean, thus ensuring that they did no further scientific work involving the use of living animals. While there is prima facie evidence that there were breaches of the Animals (Scientific Procedures) Act 1986, we consider that, in the light of all the circumstances of the case, including the effective administrative action already taken, no further purpose would be served by asking the Director of Public Prosecutions to consider prosecution."

The Committee endorses this decision which brings to an end consideration of those matters particular to the Feldberg affair. The Committee will however continue to monitor whether the general lessons to be learnt from this serious case have been learnt and acted upon.'

The first actual prosecution of a scientist under the A(SP)A occurred in 1998. Details of the case appeared in the Scottish newspaper, *The Herald*, in July 1998.

A 55-year-old Research Fellow of the University of Glasgow Vet School, pleaded guilty to breaching the A(SP)A by applying doses of deadly parasites to a herd of Friesian cows without a proper government licence.

He also admitted carrying out the experiment without a relevant certificate of designation for the land on which the experiments were performed.

The court heard that 45 cows worth an estimated £35,000 died during his project. His plea of not guilty to wilfully injecting the beasts with an injurious substance was accepted. He did hold a Home Office licence for the study of parasites. It applied only to cattle on land owned by the university.

He had 90 cattle artificially infected with lung worm and gut worm parasites. It was claimed that his intent was not to cause disease, but to infect the ground to ensure sufficient naturally acquired parasites for later experiments.

When animals began to die no remedial action was taken, but other beasts were added to the project. The cause of death in most cases was acute bacterial pneumonia.

In passing a sentence of 120 hours of community service the Sheriff, John Fitzsimons, stressed: 'I am not dealing with a case of deliberate cruelty to animals.' He added: 'What makes this such a serious case is the fact that he did not call in a vet when it became clear that something was wrong – and that even after the RSPCA had contacted the authorities, more cattle were introduced to the experiment.'

Even where there is doubt that an offence has been committed involving more than a technical breach, consideration will be given to referring the matter to the Crown Prosecution Service. While a decision to refer a case to the Crown Prosecution Service is made by the Home Office, the decision to prosecute is made by the Crown Prosecution Service alone, based on judgement of the merits of the case, the evidence available and other relevant factors, including whether a prosecution would be in the public interest. In Northern Ireland and Scotland this legal process varies as regards the governmental departments involved. With devolution very much to the fore in political circles, it might be appropriate to note the relevant websites.

Infringements and non-criminal sanctions

Most infringements, which can vary from the merely technical to the very serious, come to light through the vigilance of the Home Office Inspectors.

A document issued by the Home Office – 'Handling of infringements' – clarified the Home Office system of dealing with breaches of the Act and terms and conditions on licences.

Handling of infringements

Introduction

It is a requirement of s. 18(2)(e) of the Animals (Scientific Procedures) Act 1986 that inspectors report all infringements of the Act and of the terms and conditions of licences and certificates – however minor – to the Secretary of State along with a recommendation for the action to be taken.

Class 1

Class 1 infringements will include very minor infringements for which formal admonition, or variation, or revocation of authorities are clearly not necessary; which are not classed under ss. 22 or 23 of the Act as offences; and which do not have any animal welfare consequences. It is difficult to give definitive examples because assessment of the severity of the infringement must depend on a variety of factors. However, such infringements might include inadequate cage labelling, or failure to submit on time a report requested by licence conditions.

Inspectors will be able to deal with these infringements themselves, either verbally or in writing. However, to fulfil the requirements of s. 18(2)(e), the infringement must be reported on file and drawn to the attention of the local Animal Procedures Section caseworker, with a recommendation that no further action be taken. The caseworker will be free to seek advice from more senior members of the Animal Procedures Section if they have any concerns or doubts about the recommendation.

If the problem is not rectified, the status of the case will be raised to a higher class. Similarly, a further Class 1 infringement by the same person within five years, will automatically be treated as Class 2.

Class 2

Class 2 will cover more serious cases, but again those having no welfare consequences and for which variation or revocation of authorities is clearly not necessary. Examples might include failure to correct cage labelling when asked to do so by the Inspectorate, or a minor, accidental breach of administrative licence conditions.

In these cases, the Inspectorate will file a brief report of the circumstances. Only one recommendation can be made – a formal letter of admonition to be sent by the local caseworker. The caseworker will be required to send a copy of the report to a more senior officer in Animal Procedures Section before writing to the licensee.

If the problem is not rectified or an individual is involved in another infringement, the case will automatically be treated as Class 3.

Class 3

All other infringements (unless and until it is decided to refer the matter to the prosecuting authorities) will be treated as Class 3.

These will be handled according to the following procedures:

- The local inspector will investigate the case and provide a detailed report (setting out the circumstances and other relevant factors and making recommendations for the action to be taken) which will be attached to the relevant licence files.

- The files, with the local inspector's recommendation, will then be referred to one of the Superintending Inspectors and then to the Chief Inspector and at the same time the local caseworker will send letters notifying those involved that an infringement report has been received and that a decision will be taken within 20 working days, after which they will be informed of the outcome and their position.
- Any information provided, within those 20 days, by those involved will be taken into account in deciding what action to take.
- Concurrently, changes will be allowed to the relevant licences and certificates, with the approval of the Head of the Animal Procedures Section, but only where they do not prejudice or anticipate the outcome of the infringement.
- After consideration by the Inspectorate, the case will then be referred to the Head of the Animal Procedures Section to consider the Inspectorate's recommendation.
- Final letters will be sent advising those involved of their rights to make representations, under s. 12 of the Act, if it is proposed to revoke or vary their licence.

Reporting of infringements

All Class 1 and 2 infringements will be recorded by the local caseworker and summaries passed to more senior members of the Animal Procedures Section. All infringements will continue to be reported, retrospectively and in an anonymised form, to the Animal Procedures Committee.

An outside description of Home Office action on infringements appeared in *The Guardian* (24 June 1993). It was reported that the Home Office investigated Wickam Laboratories following infiltration by a former policeman, Neil Fry, on behalf of the British Union for the Abolition of Vivisection (BUAV).

The Home Office reported that the major allegations made by the BUAV – that animals were used unnecessarily, that there was unauthorised re-use of animals and that inadequate caging led to animal suffering – were not substantiated, but did reveal a number of weaknesses in procedures and practices. The Home Office minister, Charles Wardle, announced that he was satisfied that 'all the work carried out by Wickham was properly licensed under the Act'.

The Home Office required a number of changes to be made at Wickham to strengthen perceived weaknesses in local management practices, which led to 'a readiness to falsify' test data and 'one case of unnecessary animal use'. These changes included replacement of the named day-to-day care person, and removal of his personal licence, and improvements to formal technical training and operational procedures. The Minister said that the Medicines Control Agency considered that the faults 'did not call in question the validity of the particular tests, nor did they raise doubts about Wickham's continued operation as a contract research establishment'.

How to prevent infringements

- Always check carefully the details on certificates and licences.
- Even more carefully check the text of amendments on certificates and licences.
- Do not start work until the documents of authority are delivered to you.
- Ensure easy availability of licences and certificates so that all involved in the proposed work can personally consult them regularly, especially before commencing new procedures. Due security should of course be taken into consideration to protect the relevant documents.
- Those who work under more than one project licence must take particular care to ensure that the requisite authority is in the project which they are working under at the time.
- Make sure you are fully aware of the appropriate severity limits.
- If in doubt concerning re-use, discuss the matter with the supervisor and the inspector.
- Report any unexpected findings to the supervisor and NVS.
- Know the NACWO and consult regularly.
- Be sure that your training certificate covers the species you work with.

Note: Failure to check is no defence. 'Ignorance of the law excuses no man'. (cf. Guidance, nn. 7.14–19.)

Prosecutions under the Protection of Animals Act 1911 involving research establishments

The British Union for the Abolition of Vivisection v. *The Royal College of Surgeons* (1985) was commented upon in Chapter 1.

The case in 1989 involving a company which supplied beagles for research but unfortunately lost 79 of them en route to Sweden because of lack of the provision of adequate ventilation was also dealt with in Chapter 1.

It would not be possible to improve upon the APC's reporting of a 1997 case associating a prosecution under the 1911 Act with a research establishment.

'106. On 26 March, Channel 4 broadcast a programme entitled "It's a Dog's Life" as part of their "Countryside Undercover" series. The programme featured video material recorded in a dog toxicology unit by an undercover investigator who had worked at the establishment in the Autumn of 1996. The material showed dogs being physically abused and made other allegations about the operation of the Act at the establishment.

107. The Committee first discussed the implications of this programme at our April meeting. We were provided with an account of immediate Home Office actions. We strongly approved of the decisions to suspend immediately the personal licences of two persons shown in the film to be mistreating dogs and to refer the matter to local police to investigate possible offences under

the Protection of Animals Act 1911. We unequivocally condemned the brutality that was shown in the film and noted that these two individuals were subsequently convicted of offences under the 1911 Act. Some members expressed concern, however, about the sentences imposed by the court which they felt were too lenient.

108. At this very early point, although immediate action had been taken, the Home Office had not decided how the matter should be investigated, and indeed wished to take our views on this matter. One option put to us was that the Chief Inspector personally carry out the investigation, but we also considered an independent investigation. There were practical problems to an independent investigation: only inspectors (or the police, with a warrant) have a right of access to establishments; and it would take too long to arrange when speed of response was critical. The over-riding consideration was, however, that we had confidence in the Chief Inspector carrying out a thorough and impartial investigation. We recommended, therefore, that he proceed.

109. The Inspectorate had attracted criticism for not identifying the problems shown in the broadcast. The Committee felt this to be unfair. Even if the Inspectorate was significantly enlarged, inspectors could not be present at an establishment all the time and the sort of actions shown in the programme would never have taken place in front of an inspector. Indeed, it is extremely unlikely that any third party inspection system would have picked up the physical abuses.

110. The Chief Inspector's final report was submitted to Ministers in July. Whilst it was clear that the certificate holder had no knowledge of the problems, he was ultimately responsible to the Home Office for conduct within the establishment. It was subsequently announced, through a Parliamentary Question, that the certificate of designation would be revoked but that, to avoid the destruction of animals, the proposed revocation would be delayed for 4 months. An application for a replacement certificate would only be considered if 16 stringent conditions designed to rectify the problems identified and to prevent recurrence, had been met. These conditions are attached at Appendix D to this report.'

The conditions were met with great difficulty by Huntingdon Life Sciences.

Peripheral litigation

Animal rights activists

Since these events Huntingdon Life Sciences has continued to be targeted by SHAC (Stop Huntingdon Animal Cruelty). This pressure group has spread its aggression beyond Huntingdon, even forcing, in this century, the Institute of Animal Technology to hold their Annual Congress outside the UK.

The activities of SHAC are typical of various other pressure groups opposed to the use of animals in research and are vivid examples of the difficulties faced by research workers. It would hardly be appropriate in this book on laboratory law to list the numerous acts of terrorism perpetrated against designated establishments and the reactions of governments, but an allusion to the need for awareness of the hazards of animal experimentation is hardly out of place. This is a continuous and widespread threat not confined only to this country.

The US arm of SHAC itself was convicted, along with six activists, of inciting violence and terrorism in an attempt to shut down Huntingdon Life Sciences (HLS), Britain's largest animal testing facility, which has a branch in New Jersey. Although all the accused were American, one of the group was a key player in the movement in Britain and controlled SHAC while its British leaders were in prison.

The FBI has already claimed that animal rights extremists posed the greatest terror threat in America. The conviction is thought to be the first achieved under the animal enterprise terrorism legislation, which is similar to 'economic sabotage' laws that were introduced in Britain in the summer of 2005 and were designed specifically to combat animal rights extremism. The offences were similar to those suffered by British victims. SHAC used its website to incite threats, harassment and vandalism. The accused were convicted variously of animal enterprise terrorism and multiple counts of conspiring and committing interstate stalking and of telephone harassment. Those convicted of all three offences faced a maximum 14 years in prison and substantial fines. SHAC as an organisation was also convicted and its American website was taken down.

Coincidentally, the day before this conviction one of SHAC's founder members was jailed for breaching an anti-social behaviour order and was given a four-month prison sentence by Oxford Crown Court.

This information has been taken from *Times on Line* 04/03/2006 (http://www. timesonline.co.uk/article/0,,11069-2068837,00.html).

Government response has not always been so dramatic.

'The Halls have been driven to close their farm, which breeds guinea pigs for medical research, after a six year sustained campaign of terror by animal rights extremists. Over that time, they have been subjected to numerous death threats, a firebomb attack and hundreds of acts of criminal damage. The final straw for the Halls was the desecration of the grave and theft of the remains of one family member, Gladys Hammond [a grandmother], by a group calling itself the Animal Rights Militia.
[. . .]
When the Halls finally threw in the towel earlier this week the Government did not immediately condemn the tactics of the animal rights lobby. Staffordshire police arrested 60 protestors over the years, 28 of whom have been cautioned and charged, mostly on minor public-order offences.
[. . .]

The Government admittedly did help Huntingdon Life Sciences when no commercial bank would work with it, by offering it an account at the Bank of England instead. Yet the company was still forced to re-register in Maryland in order to keep its shareholders' home addresses private and stop them suffering the same fate as the company's chief executive, Brian Cass, who was beaten up with baseball bats outside his home.'

(Editorial, *The Spectator*, 27/8/05, p. 5)

Legal action against extremists

Violent activity against persons and property in research has always been illegal. Perpetrators of arson attacks, criminal damage and assault could always be prosecuted successfully as long as sufficient evidence could be gathered. Antivivisectionists, however, have proved to be adept at exploiting legal loopholes and indulging with impunity in aggressive protests, intimidation and harassment.

The government has strived to update legislation to deal with this menace in order to protect research establishments and those who are associated with them either as workers, suppliers, contractors or financial associates.

The Public Order Act of 1986 provided limited protection against aggressive protests. It was found necessary in 2003 to strengthen the impact of this law by amending the definition of an assembly of persons from 20 to 2.

The Malicious Communications Act 1988 was amended in the Criminal Justice and Police Act 2001 to cover electronic communications in order to close an emerging legal loophole. Penalties were also increased.

Similarly the Criminal Justice and Public Order Act 1994 in 2003 applied aggravated trespass to buildings as well as to open-air protests.

The Criminal Justice and Police Act 2001 also amended the Protection from Harassment Act 1997 so that it became an offence to aid, abet, counsel or procure another person to carry out harassment. This was a move to remove immunity of prosecution from those who had safely directed the foot soldiers from afar.

The Prevention of Terrorism Act 2000 by widening the definition of terrorism provided greater scope for the police to apply this law to animal rights extremists.

The Criminal Justice and Public Order Act 2001 gave the police new powers to direct protestors away from homes and introduced changes to the Companies Act allowing company directors to use service addresses rather than home addresses on the Companies House register.

The serious Organised Crime and Police Act 2005 enables the police to deal with animal rights extremists more effectively, especially through the 'economic damage' clause.

While the written law in this area appeared adequate, to some in the scientific field the enforcement of relevant legislation seemed wanting to a certain extent. Now the National Extremism Tactical Coordination Unit (NETCU) provides guidance to all police forces, so it is hoped that the application of the above Acts will be patently effective.

Antivivisectionists' use of the law

My first contact with the British Union for the Abolition of Vivisection (BUAV) was in 1985 in a drawn-out case at the magistrates' court in Bromley and later at the Crown court in Croydon. The BUAV were unsuccessful in their attempt to prosecute the Royal College of Surgeons. The case is referred to in Chapter 1. The BUAV have specialised in pursuing their antivivisectionist cause by legal means and continually press for a rigorous application of the A(SP)A. Their ultimate aim is to end animal experimentation by:

- peacefully campaigning and lobbying to change laws and government policies
- challenging negative perceptions around animal rights
- providing information on and raising awareness of animal experimentation.
  (email: info@buav.org) (cf. http://www.buav.org/)

Soon after the 1998 amendment of A(SP)A, the BUAV legally challenged the Home Office, claiming that the amended s. 5(5) no longer allowed the licensing of the LD50 test if a suitable non-animal or less aggressive protocol is available, claiming that there were such alternative protocols for LD50. The Home Office took the view, following legal advice, that it would no longer grant licences if a suitable alternative was available. The Department held by its view that LD50 tests which are aimed simply at meeting the regulatory requirements of a foreign jurisdiction and which have no other scientific justification, can no longer be said to meet the terms of s. 5 (cf. Home Office statement, 21/11/99, n. 115).

In 2001 the BUAV again threatened the Home Office with judicial review proceedings for not completely outlawing the use of mice in the production of monoclonal antibodies by the ascites method. The BUAV also claimed that the Home Office was bound to forbid the use of a painful skin sensitisation test involving guinea pigs which should be completely replaced by an alternative LLNA (local lymph node assay). The LLNA had been validated by the European Centre for the Validation of Alternative Methods (ECVAM). The Home Office pointed out that it was observing s. 5 of the A(SP)A by outlawing unnecessary use of the ascites method and that the LLNA may not be suitable for pharmaceutical products (cf. *RDS News*, October 2001, p. 2).

Most prominent among the various legal ventures of the BUAV in recent times, (i.e. 2006), has been a prolonged attempt to obtain a judicial review against the Home Office on the following grounds:

- On the classification of severity limits and bandings applied to animal research.
- On the provisions of monitoring and care of animals at Cambridge University.
- On the use of the repetitive testing of marmosets in small Perspex boxes at Cambridge University.
- Whether the welfare of stock animals should be taken into consideration in the cost/benefit analyses under the Act.
- Whether the death of an animal is an 'adverse effect' within the Act and therefore has to be taken into account when the decision to grant a licence is taken.

- Whether guidelines on food and water restrictions should have been produced as a code of practice, and thus taken through the process laid down for
such codes.

On 12/04/05 BUAV were granted permission to seek judicial review only on
the last two points: whether the death of an animal is an 'adverse effect' and whether
the guidelines on food and water is a code of practice. The judge rejected the BUAV's
arguments about severity limits and all the points relating to Cambridge University.

The BUAV persisted in their questioning of the treatment of animals at
Cambridge University. On 18/07/05 the organisation was granted, on appeal,
permission to seek judicial reviews on two more of the above points: the use of the
marmosets and monitoring of the animals. The prolonged controversy continues (2007).

The impact of the Freedom of Information Act (FOI)

Many in research work are concerned about the application of the FOI (www.
homeoffice.gov.uk/about-us/freedom-of-information) in view of the behaviour of
some antivivisectionists.

In a press release on 01/01/05 the BUAV have already suggested that the Home
Office would not fully implement the terms of the FOI as regards applications for
project licences. The press release implies that the Home Office is producing a
smoke screen by stressing the significance of the 'abstract' while retaining the secrecy
of the full details of the project. The BUAV maintains that the FOI renders the
confidentiality clause in legislation governing animal experimentation redundant
(http://www.buav.org/press/2005/01.html).

In keeping with the recommendations of the Select Committee on Animals in
Scientific Procedures issued by the House of Lords (16/07/02), some abstracts attached
to project licence applications were released into the public domain in 2005. Now
in 2007 there are 100s of abstracts on the HO website.

The FOI gives anybody the right to access information held by public authorities, including central government departments. It is difficult to foresee future effects
of this Act in the area of research. Decisions on freedom of information are case
by case, so there are no sweeping exemptions for any types of document. It is,
therefore, always wise to mark any of your written work which you regard as
sensitive 'CONFIDENTIAL'. This could not apply, of course, to the above-mentioned
abstract, but would probably be an appropriate stipulation as regards most of the
rest of the information involved in an application for a project licence. In this
context there is also the Data Protection Act 1998 which requires that sufficient
security measures are in place to safeguard against unauthorised or unlawful
accessing and/or processing of personal data.

Personal information is exempt from disclosure. Commercial companies are not
themselves subject to the FOI. However, information held on their behalf at the
Home Office would be.

A letter from the Home Office (22/04/05) to certificate holders on current
practice under the FOI is informative and to a certain extent reassuring.

'Up to the end of March we have received seventeen requests for information relating to the production and use of animals for experimentation and other scientific purposes. Of these, four were from journalists, eight from NGOs, and five from members of the public. The information requested has included the contents of inspection reports, details of project licences, names of individuals, companies and academic institutions licensed under the 1986 Act, and information about the importation of non-human primates to the UK.

To date we have answered thirteen of these requests, providing some fairly basic, non-sensitive information. No information has been provided about individuals working under the Act. Also in handling a request for information contained in project licences for which abstracts have been published on the Home Office website, we concluded that there was little additional information to disclose beyond what was already provided in the well-constructed abstracts.

From these early cases, it appears that the FOI provides adequate safeguards for the information we hold, although none of our decisions have yet been tested through the appeal process available to applicants.

Section 38 has been relevant to most requests, as have Sections 40, 41 and 44. Section 43 hasn't figured much, yet Section 12 applied in two cases where the cost of providing the information requested would have exceeded the £600 limit applicable to Government Departments (the limit for other public bodies in England and Wales is £450).'

An article in the *RDS News*, January 2004, p. 7, has an apt comment on the confidentiality theme. It points out that although released material may be fully anonymised, interested campaigners could obtain information on a particular area of work by using the correct key words on the internet. Extremists successfully traced scientists working with guinea pigs all over the country without any FOI.

The FOI covers England, Wales and Northern Ireland (the text can be viewed at: http://www.hmso.gov.uk/acts/2000/20000036.htm). The Freedom of Information (Scotland) Act is a similar piece of legislation (www.opsi.gov.uk/legislation/scotland/acts2002/20020013.htm).

Procedures for making representations

The Statutory Instrument 1986 No. 1911 (Animals) laid down the Rules for appeal against a decision of the Secretary of State involving use of animals in research, for example revocation or varying of conditions on a licence or certificate. The details of the order are couched in legal jargon but are expounded fully in Guidance Appendix H accompanied by the text of the Statutory Instrument in Guidance Annex to Appendix H. Points to note are:

- One should notify the Secretary of State of one's intention to make representation.
- A legally qualified person will be appointed to consider any such representation.

- The Secretary of State will send lists and copies of all relevant documents to him/her and to the person considering the case.
- One has the right to opt for an oral or written form of representation and even for a public hearing.
- One may call witnesses, address the person appointed and be represented at the hearing.
- If an Inspector's report is involved one may question the Inspector who made the report.

Before embarking on such a process of appeal one should refer to Guidance Appendix H and preferably seek the advice of a legal expert in the field.

It was nearly 20 years before this first Statutory Instrument of the Act, SI 1986, No. 1911, was fully implemented in the form of a public tribunal headed by a QC, in March 2005. This was the first direct challenge to the Home Secretary by a project licence applicant. Crucial though this unique case was, it was surprisingly low key in its performance. On one day of the hearing, the expected public was represented solely by myself. On the other few days of the process there was a marked absence of groups who would have been presumed to be interested parties, even 'stakeholders'.

Professor Twink Allen of the Equine Fertility Unit in Newmarket had applied to the Home Office in 2001 for a project licence to implant cloned embryos into female horses. He made a case to clone embryos to produce high-performing sport horses. In his application, he pointed out that it is difficult to breed dressage, show jumping, eventing, endurance and carriage-driving horses, and polo ponies, because many star performers are geldings.

A BBC correspondent, Christine McGourty, reported in BBC News (05/05/04, 7.12 a.m.) that the Home Office had spent several years examining the issue before concluding that the benefits did not outweigh the possible costs to the animal involved. Professor Allen appealed against the decision when the Home Office rejected his application because of concerns about animal welfare. The fact that Italian scientists had successfully cloned a horse for the first time in August 2003 acted as a spur to Professor Allen's endeavours. He further argued that his technique would be a method of selecting superior males and females to produce better genetic stock and would be a 'quantum leap forward'. He told the House of Lords Select Committee in 2002 that he did not see any 'ethical or welfare' considerations arising from his intended project.

On 30/03/05 *The Guardian* (p. 4) announced a Home Office decision to allow an application for a project licence by Professor Allen to clone horses for research purposes. The permission would be granted subject to regular progress reports being provided to the Home Office, including details of any welfare costs it might entail. There was to be no doubt that the ban on the cloning of horses for purely commercial reasons, such as the cloning of champion racehorses, remains.

Professor Allen told *The Guardian* newspaper: 'I'm very pleased, but disappointed they haven't gone the whole hog and allowed us sensibly to clone for commercial reasons, where there is a real need for it. The value of the cloning would be to create the champion gelding, or at least his testicles [sic].'

The *Horse and Hound Online* (*01/04/05*) provides the Parthian shot. 'However, Timothy Corner QC, who advised the government on the matter, didn't rule out commercial cloning forever and wrote in his report that "if in the future there is produced either evidence of greater benefit [of cloning] than I have identified, or evidence that the costs are less, then a different view might be taken".'

In my opinion it would be difficult to find a more perfect summing-up of the spirit of the A(SP)A in practice than the last statement.

Chapter 14

Officials and Committees

Home Office Inspectors

Inspectors must have the veterinary or medical qualifications demanded by the Secretary of State and all have higher academic or professional qualifications and experience of various forms of research in the life sciences. The number of inspectors has gradually increased over the years. A target of 33 has been mentioned. They are committed to visiting about 230 widely separated establishments, with a target to visit every place, however small or inaccessible, at least once a year. These visits are made from regional offices in London, Swindon, Shrewsbury, Dundee and Cambridge. Northern Ireland is the responsibility of the Department of Health and Social Services of Northern Ireland. A close relationship exists between the Inspectorate and the inspector who serves Northern Ireland. The Inspectorate is part of the Animals Scientific Procedures Division of the Science and Research Group in the Home Office and works closely with the Licensing and Policy Sections of the Division.

According to the A(SP)A (s. 18(2)) the statutory duties of the Inspector are:

- 'to advise the Secretary of State on applications for certificates and licences, on requests for their variation or revocation and, in the case of personal licences, on their periodical review;
- to visit places where regulated procedures are carried out to check whether those procedures are authorized by the necessary licences and whether the conditions of those licences are being complied with;
- to visit scientific procedure, breeding and supplying establishments for the purpose of determining whether the conditions of the certificates in respect of those establishments are being complied with and;
- to report to the Secretary of State any case in which any provision of this Act or any condition of a licence or certificate under the Act has not been or is not being complied with, and to advise on the action to be taken on any such case.'

The inspector has the executive power to require that an animal which he/she considers is undergoing excessive suffering be immediately killed in an appropriate manner.

An inspector has an important role in identifying and disseminating best welfare and scientific practice, providing operational and professional insights into policy development, implementation, maintenance and review. The comprehensive role of the inspector can be summed up in the four terms – advice, review, inspect and report.

The prominent function of the inspectors for most research workers is their role as assessors of proposals in applications for certificates and licences. Inspectors are the primary assessors and it is their duty to assess in detail and challenge where necessary, to determine whether the likely benefits outweigh the cost in the suffering of the animals to be used. They must question if there is more scope for the 3Rs. To make these judgements they need to be fully aware of the scientific quality and validity of the proposed work, the appropriateness of the animal use and the measures taken to minimise animal suffering. Such investigation, to be productive, requires frank discussion in detail with applicants. Having come to a decision based on the results of this challenging of an applicant, the inspectors offer their professional advice to the Secretary of State on whether, and on what terms, the application should be granted. The inspector may advise applications for licences or amendments be referred to external assessors or the APC. Internal consultation within the Inspectorate is common.

In the case of designated establishments the inspector monitors standards and encourages good practice. The inspector will report non-compliance with the conditions of designation and any other breaches discovered during inspections which may be made without notice. The inspector should be given ready access to any area of a designated establishment. The inspector has a reasonable right of entry to designated establishments, as noted in Chapter 9 in respect to the responsibility of the CH. Absolute legal right of entry is ruled by s. 25 of the A(SP)A which involves a constable with a warrant of entry, and if the place is a designated establishment the constable is required to be accompanied by a Home Office inspector (cf. Guidance Appendix G, nn. 7–17).

In 2000 the Code for Licensing and Inspection was replaced by a Charter on Licensing and Inspection (see Chapter 10).

A specific stipulation of the Charter is concerned with the availability of inspectors for discussion and advice, a valuable contribution to the smooth working of the project licensing system. In this context the perennial contention concerning the variation of inspectoral opinions arises. Even the APC saw fit to comment on this phenomenon which naturally occurs when different individuals comment on the interpretation of rules not actually etched in stone.

> 'Such is the variety of designated places and research proposals, however, that a flexible response is essential to match advice precisely to local circumstances. Thus it is consistency rather than uniformity which is sought. Similar proposals and facilities are seldom identical in practice. It should not come as a surprise that similar applications, once all the relevant factors are weighed (including the experience of the personnel involved, their track record, and the resources available), result in differing advice to the Secretary of State by the Inspectorate.'

(APC Report 1997, p. 63, nn. 2–5)

Other Home Office civil servants are involved in the administration of the A(SP)A. They process the licensing system. It is staff in the Animal Procedures Section that grant, refuse, vary, revoke and suspend licences and certificates for the Secretary of State. They also administer the collection of fees. (cf. Guidance Appendix G, nn. 4 and 5.)

In Northern Ireland the Department of Health, Social Services and Public Safety administers the Act.

In October of 2005 a welcome development appeared in the form of an Animals (Scientific Procedures) Inspectorate Annual Report 2004, distinct from the APC Annual Report and in addition to the annual publication of Statistics of Scientific Procedures on Animals. It provides a valuable insight into the work done by inspectors and how the inspectorate arrives at its decisions. It addresses the three prominent problems which I encounter in 5th modules for applicants for project licences.

Could the recommendations of inspectors be comparable and consistent?

> 'With nearly thirty inspectors of differing backgrounds, it is important to promote the application of common principles and comparable standards. This does not mean working to a rigid set of rules, but applying a set of principles to each different situation, so that in identical circumstances the actions or recommendations of different inspectors would be comparable and consistent. The importance of such consistency is emphasised during the initial training of new inspectors, and the many informal discussions between inspectors, joint visiting, and the movement of responsibility for places between inspectors approximately every five years all help maintain consistency. There are regional office and national discussions of cases, and quarterly national meetings specifically to look at consistency. For certain matters special interest inspectors provide a national source of advice, and the half-yearly inspectors' conferences provide opportunities to exchange views and consider particular topics.'
>
> (p. 8)

How long does it take to get a project licence?

> 'The Inspectorate aims to assess proposals for new work so that those authorities which can be recommended are in place by the time the applicants need them. This is to avoid wastage of animals on continuing programmes of work, missing of key dates for progress of new medicine developments, or delaying time-dependent funded programmes. In addition for the last few years [written in 2005] inspectors have worked with licensing staff to a target of 35 working days for processing within the Home Office of 85% of new project applications' (page 10).

In practice it appears that most applications for personal licences are usually processed within a month.

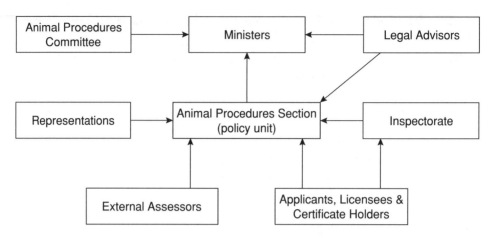

Fig. 14.1   Home Office Responsibilities

Is the confidential information supplied in an application for a project licence protected?

> 'The Inspectorate's Annual Report contributes to the Government's commitment to openness by giving more information on the work of the Inspectorate than has been previously available, for example, in the commentary of the annual publication of Statistics of Scientific Procedures on Living Animals. Future reports are expected to feature material prepared by inspectors that has previously been provided as contributions to the annual reports of the Animal Procedures Committee. Care has been taken in this report to anonymise examples and preserve confidentiality, conscious that the 1986 Act prohibits the unauthorized disclosure of confidential material.' [cf. comment on the Freedom of Information Act in Chapter 13 of this text.]

> 'It is also sadly necessary to safeguard places and personnel (including inspectors) against the activities of animal rights extremists. For this reason no names or location details are included in the report and confidential information or anything that might identify places or individuals has been omitted' (page 2).

'Other staff in the Section are responsible for providing advice on or replies to correspondence concerning the use of animals in scientific procedures and for providing support to Ministers on policy issues relating to the Act.'

(Guidance Appendix G, p. 89, Fig. 14.1)

The Animal Procedures Committee (APC)

This proactive committee is an independent advisory body established by the A(SP)A (ss. 19 and 20) to provide strategic advice to the Secretary of State on policy, practice, ethics, science and welfare. It 'shall have regard both to the legitimate requirements of science and unnecessary use in scientific procedures' (s. 20(2)). The APC is kept informed of infringements of the Act.

The minimum membership is 12 and a Chairman. Two-thirds of the members must be medical practitioners or veterinary surgeons, or qualified or experienced in a biological subject. One member must be a barrister, solicitor or advocate. At least half of the members must not currently hold, or have held within the past six years, any licence under the Act. Members are appointed by the Secretary of State on personal merit. They do not represent interest groups. The maximum tenure is two periods of two years.

In 1998 the APC produced a Code of Conduct for its members (cf. Guidance Appendix G, nn. 19–36).

One of the salient functions of the APC is in its role as a consultant body to the Secretary of State on the issuing of licences in particular sensitive categories of research. The types of licence applications which are referred for consideration to the APC are to be found in the 2005 Application for a Project Licence form at p. 2, section 15. Referral to the APC occurs if the proposed project involves:

- non-human primates, dogs, cats or equidae in substantial protocols
- wild-caught non-human primates
- xenotransplantation of whole organs if the whole project is in the substantial severity band or there are major animal welfare or ethical concerns
- chronic pain and/or central nervous studies if the whole project is in the substantial severity band or there are major animal welfare or ethical concerns.

Applications raising novel policy issues or other concerns may also be referred to the APC.

Advice on this matter is given in the notes accompanying the Application for a Project Licence (p. 5, n. 15) and 'You are advised to consult a Home Office Inspector on the preparation of such applications.'

According to information given by the Home Office Minister, Caroline Flint MP, to Parliament and the APC in 2004, these other concerns include contentious issues or applications giving rise to serious societal concerns. (As an example, this would include any application involving the genetic modification of non-human primates or embryo aggregation chimaeras involving dissimilar species.)

The Minister took this opportunity to stress that referred applications should not be unduly delayed. The APC at their meeting on 9 February 2005 discussed a *modus operandi* of a proposed Applications Sub-Committee to expedite the procedure. The APC played a leading part in the ending of the use of animals in testing cosmetics in this country.

The 1996 APC Report deals with this topic at some length and justifiably comments:

> 'Consideration of applications to test cosmetic products or ingredients on animals is one of the most difficult aspects of our work and always provokes intense and wide ranging discussion.'
>
> (p. 5, n. 43)

Other relevant extracts concerning cosmetics are:

'No new applications for cosmetic testing licences were considered during 1996.'

(p. 5, n. 45)

'. . . the 6th Council Amendment to the European Cosmetic Directive which sought to ban the marketing of cosmetics tested on animals after 1 January 1998 (but only if validated alternative tests are in place). However, it was already clear in 1996 that validated alternatives for tests would not be in place and that the proposed ban would, therefore, be postponed by the European Union.'

(p. 5, n. 47)

There is an intriguing comment in n. 48 on the same page which refers to controversy concerning the testing of other products which could be considered to be 'unnecessary'. No details are given.

'The Act required that programmes of work are authorized on a case-by-case basis. The Act itself prohibits no particular type of procedures – such as the use of animals in the testing of cosmetic products. This is a disappointment to many critics but it exemplifies the point made in the Committee's report that the law provides a framework in which to balance the likely costs to animals against the benefits to man, animals or the environment.'

(p. 36, n. 8)

The sensitive nature and importance of this topic is apparent from the serious comment on the above material which appeared in the *LASA Newsletter* (Winter 1997).

'A further response was issued by the Home Office on 6 November 1997 to announce that it had made further progress on the matter. It said that an end to cosmetic products testing, which was being sought when the Home Secretary's response was published had now been secured. The three companies undertaking this type of work in the UK had voluntarily agreed to stop cosmetic products testing. Current licences were being amended to prohibit such testing.

Legal advice had been taken and confirmed that revocation of current licences was not possible under the Animals (Scientific Procedures) Act 1986. A voluntary agreement was therefore the quickest way to achieve the cessation of cosmetics testing. An outright ban is not possible without primary legislation (this would seem to be beyond the scope of the enabling process associated with the ASPA, allowing for secondary legislation through Statutory Instruments), but the Government will issue no new licences for the testing of finished cosmetic products on animals.

The Government also stated that it wished to see an end to the testing of ingredients used in certain forms of cosmetics which can be called vanity products. The definition of these products and the differentiation of their ingredients from others will need the advice of the APC and consultation with interest groups and industry. The difficulties arise because the ingredients of some vanity products are also used in a variety of other commodities where safety testing is regarded as essential including some pharmaceutical products.'

It is important to recall the official definition of 'cosmetic' contained in a former European Community Directive (76/768) on this subject:

'Any substance or preparation intended for placing in contact with the various parts of the human body (epidermis, hair system, nails, lips and external genital organs) or with the teeth and mucous membranes of the oral cavity with a view exclusively or principally to cleaning them, perfuming them or protecting them, in order to keep them in good condition, change their appearance or correct body odours.'

It is this definition that is followed for the purposes of the Act (cf. former edition of HOG Q. 17). It is obvious that in this context 'cosmetic' is not just the latest perfumery accessory but includes 'down-to-earth' soap.

The *LASA Newsletter* (Winter 1997) adds a further significant comment:

'The Government will also take the opportunity to explore, at the same time, the feasibility of a ban on testing finished household products on animals.'

The definitive statement on animal use in the testing of cosmetics aptly appeared among other important material in the APC 1998 Report (p. 2):

'16. The Government made some significant announcements in November. These included:
– an end to the use of animals in the testing of cosmetics ingredients, secured through a voluntary agreement with the companies carrying out this type of work in the UK – this was in addition to the end to finished products testing announced in 1997;
– agreement that this Committee should be, and be seen to be, more independent and proactive. This would be facilitated by the setting up of a dedicated secretariat; and
– the appointment of new members to the Committee.'

The Winter 1997 *LASA Newsletter* also indicated the trend as regards other tests using animals:

'The Government will not allow tests which involve animals in the development and testing of alcohol or tobacco products. At present no such licences exist and none will be authorized in the future.'

APC comments on cloning

In keeping with its more proactive role which has evolved, especially during the 1990s, the APC produced an interesting commentary on the development of cloning, with particular reference to the ovine milestone, Dolly.

'115. In February 1997, articles appeared in the press announcing that scientists at the Roslin Institute had bred a lamb called Dolly, produced through a revolutionary cloning process.

116. In part, the cloning process had followed a well-established method whereby the nucleus of an egg cell is removed. The distinctive aspect of the new process that led to Dolly was that the replacement nucleus (to form the embryo) was that of a specialised cell from an adult animal. The specialised cell had been persuaded to return to a state of quiescence in which it could function as a stem cell. In the past, while nuclear transfer had been commonly used, the nuclear material had always been derived from non-specialised tissue.

117. Much of the work carried out at the Roslin Institute did not need licence authority under the Animals (Scientific Procedures) Act 1986. The production of a living animal (or a foetus which was to be allowed to survive past the half-gestation period) does, however, require such authorities. The objectives of the programme, as identified in the project licence, were to create a better understanding of the biology of embryonic maturation and development, to use that knowledge to solve current welfare problems associated with established artificial breeding techniques, and to develop new and improved methods of artificial breeding applicable to agricultural animals. Other objectives included the production and rapid multiplication of transgenic agricultural animals as sources of pharmaceutical proteins and models of disease.

118. We had the opportunity to discuss this work at the March meeting of the Committee. We agreed that there were animal welfare implications to be considered in principle under the cost/benefit assessment. But the work also fell within the remit of other Government Departments, such as the Ministry of Agriculture, Fisheries and Food (which funded some of the work at Roslin). The regulatory implications of human cloning fell to the Human Fertility and Embryology Authority and the Human Genetics Advisory Committee to consider, who were clear that human cloning was forbidden in the UK.

119. There was some concern, nevertheless, that the possibility of human cloning should have been considered when the project licence had been assessed and granted. It was apparent, however, that the scientific focus had been on the immediate achievement of the study objectives. The longer term consequences and benefits had been seen as agricultural or pharmaceutical. Some members were nevertheless concerned that a potential disbenefit, of which human cloning was a good example, should be taken into account when considering costs and benefits.'

(1997 APC Report, p. 16)

APC comments on xenotransplantation

The APC discussed the responsibility of the HO apropos the significant progress in scientific research and its impact on the acceptability of xenotransplantation. Because of its importance the topic of xenotransplantation – the use of the organs of animals in humans – became the special concern of the Kennedy Commission which recommended the establishment of the UKXIRA (United Kingdom Xenotransplantation Interim Regulatory Authority). The relationship between the Home Office's operation of the A(SP)A and the scope of the UKXIRA had been considered by the APC. The Home Office is responsible for any animals used but not for determining or checking whether the quality of the animals was acceptable for use as a source of organs for clinical use. The Home Office has produced a new code of practice for the housing of high health status source animals (QPF – Qualified Pathogen Free) for transplantation. It was agreed that the Home Office would not consider project licence applications to use animals in clinical trials unless these had been endorsed by the Department of Health and UKXIRA (cf. APC Report 1997, p. 14).

Legal control of xenotransplantation continues to be an issue, well outside the scope of A(SP)A and well beyond the confines of the UK. An updating of the state of concern about this pursuit appeared in the *Veterinary Record* (14/05/06). It indicates possible trends of future legislation.

'A revised action plan to control and regulate the practice of xenotransplantation has been issued by the World Health Organization (WHO) following a recent meeting of an advisory panel of international experts.

The revised action plan includes;

- updating a compendium of guidelines and recommendations for national health authorities and regulatory bodies to deal with xenotransplantation;
- improving methods for the collection and dissemination of information on xenotransplantation practices; and
- raising greater awareness among national health authorities and promoting high ethical standards and well regulated practices.

Explaining why stricter controls are needed, the WHO points out that the main risk posed by xenotransplantation is the transmission of diseases to humans from animals. To manage this risk, several countries have developed rigorous guidelines and oversight procedures for the performance of xenotransplantation. Guidelines on xenotransplantation and its regulation are available on the WHO website: www.who.int/transplantation/xeno'

Other committees associated with A(SP)A

The House of Lords Select Committee on Animals in Scientific Procedures published its report on 24 July 2002. This committee, a branch of the legislature, sat for over a year taking evidence from a very wide range of individuals and organisations, including scientists and antivivisectionists.

The committee concluded that animal experimentation is morally acceptable and that there is a continuing need to use animals in medical research and safety testing. Its recommendations fell into three categories: efficient regulation, openness and transparency, and, of course, the 3Rs. On efficient regulation, the recommendation includes shorter, simpler project licences, giving LERPs the power to approve routine or minor amendments and allowing visiting scientists to work under their host's project licence. The last point is one I would certainly endorse.

The committee identifies other areas which might be considered: the promotion of the 3Rs in toxicology, periodic review of inspectors, the inspection of designated establishments at least annually by an inspector from another area, the relaxation of restrictions on the use of terminally anaesthetised animals for training surgeons, and the development of a scoring system to elucidate animal suffering by NVSs and NACWOs.

The committee has strong recommendations about openness, even discussing the repeal of s. 24 (the confidentiality section) of the A(SP)A. The suggested publication of substantive anonymised details of project licences has in part been met particularly as regards the wide dissemination of 'abstracts'. The following proposals were more acceptable to many research workers: a regular forum to discuss specific issues, under the auspices of the APC, Home Office statistics that are easier to interpret and better information on animal suffering.

The RDS comment was indeed apt.

> 'RDS welcomes this extremely sensible and realistic report that should be used as the blueprint for future government policy and regulation of animal research and testing.'
>
> (cf. RDS Email Service 24/07/02)

Some of the ideals of the committee are already in place, for example, the Inter-Department Group on the 3Rs.

The full text of the report is available at http://www.publications.parliament.uk/pa/ldanimal.htm

The Local Ethical Review Committee is a natural outcrop from the LERP. These committees, local by definition, do, however, constitute one of the most potent forces influencing the application of the ethical aspects of the A(SP)A (cf. Chapter 9).

Various groups have been used by the Home Office to improve the impact of the A(SP)A; for example, in 1999 the Expert Group on Efficient Regulation, under Professor Purchase as Chair, brought together experts in the operation of the animal procedure legislation with representatives of science, industry and animal welfare interest groups. The aim was to consider whether there are ways in which the administrative burden which the legislation produces could be simplified or reduced.

In October 2001 EGER issued their final report. It did not suggest any changes in legislation but delivered recommendations to the Home Office concerning aspects of administration and to certificate holders suggesting the improvement of organisation and training within establishments.

Both the Inter-Departmental Data Sharing Group (2000) and the Inter-Departmental Group on the 3Rs (2002) have been referred to in Chapter 7.

A Statistics Working Group was set up by the APC in June 2003. The Group issued a consultation document (30/11/03) on the matter to a large number of individuals. Opinions were sought not only on the nature of the statistics that should be collected regarding the use of animals under the A(SP)A but also concerning methods of presentation. The outcome of this exercise could radically affect the nature of paperwork involved in returns and applications. In the same month of 2003 the APC set up another working group to consider the issue of severity bands. This venture is discussed in Chapter 7. Both these endeavours are ongoing processes (2007).

The Home Office encourages and organises gatherings of stakeholders, especially of certificate holders, to discuss the administration of the Act and to provide the opportunity to ask questions about its application. Inspectors attend these ad hoc meetings.

An early attempt to involve stakeholders in a discussion body concerning the A(SP)A was announced in a Home Office PCD circular 2/99.

A welcome development in bringing the working of the A(SP)A before the public was announced in the Home Office PCD circular 2/99:

> 'A Forum is being organised at which scientists, animal welfarists, anti-vivisectionists and representatives of Government can discuss issues surrounding the use of animals in scientific procedures.'

Those who seek to further their aims by violence, intimidation or other such activities have not been invited. The objective of the event is:

> 'For the Minister [on behalf of the Home Office and his colleagues] to hear the range of views, to encourage open and constructive dialogue, and to identify common ground concerning the use of animals in scientific procedures.'

This was intended to be a one-off event in the first instance, but it could be repeated. The Forum was not intended to compete with the continuing work and role of the Boyd Group in seeking consensus on the way forward among the range of views concerning the use of animals in scientific procedures.

The above paragraphs feature the more important official and semi-official bodies associated with the A(SP)A. There is no doubt that other committees contributing to the development of the A(SP)A will continue to be assembled. Subcommittees of the APC do tend to proliferate. Interested parties should take cognisance of their recommendations because they may eventually, as in the past, become more than mere suggestions.

Part III

Other Relevant Legislation

Chapter 15

The Law on Veterinary Surgery

The Veterinary Surgeons Act 1966

The Act restricts the practice of veterinary surgery to specifically qualified individuals. Those permitted by law to practise veterinary surgery are persons registered as members of the Royal College of Veterinary Surgeons (RCVS). There was a closed list of qualified individuals who were entitled to practise by virtue of experience as veterinary practitioners. Apart from veterinary degrees from UK universities, holders of certain Commonwealth and South African veterinary degrees are recognised for registration. The Veterinary Surgeons Qualifications (EEC Recognition Order) 1980 recognises EEC veterinary qualifications as sufficient for the practice of veterinary surgery in this country. There was later a similar statutory instrument, Veterinary Surgeons Qualifications (European Recognition) Order 2003 No. 2919. Other relevant statutory instruments are the Veterinary Surgeons and Veterinary Practitioners (Registration) (Amendment) Regulations Order of Council 2006 No. 3255. Relevant statutory instruments are issued occasionally updating the requirements as regards veterinary qualifications. Veterinary qualified persons outside the scope of the above legislation can sit an examination set by the RCVS to obtain the necessary qualification to practise here.

A veterinary surgeon may need an owner's consent to treat an animal in order to avoid an action for trespass to goods. In case of an accident or when an animal is suffering excessively a police constable, under the Protection of Animals Act 1911, could authorise a veterinary surgeon to kill the animal without the consent of the owner. The constable's decision will be taken on the basis of a veterinary surgeon's certificate.

Veterinary surgery

The Act defines the work which is restricted to veterinary surgeons as the art and science of veterinary surgery and medicine. This definition extends to:

(a) the diagnosis of diseases in, and injuries to, animals including tests performed on animals for diagnostic purposes
(b) the giving of advice based upon such diagnosis

(c)   the medical and surgical treatment of animals

(d)   the performance of surgical operations on animals.

Anaesthesia prior to veterinary treatment is covered by the Veterinary Surgeons Act 1966, whereas that used solely for management or handling is not considered veterinary surgery and such anaesthesia may be carried out by a non-veterinarian. A veterinary surgeon carrying out anaesthesia as a regulated procedure must be authorised under the A(SP)A 1986.

Permitted treatment of animals by a lay person

(a)   Any treatment given to an animal by its owner or his employee, a member of the owner's household or his employee.

It is worth noting that the Act refers to 'any treatment' which, it might be argued, refers to item (c) above in connection with the definition of veterinary surgery and does not extend to other aspects of the definition such as diagnosis and surgical operations.

An organisation which owns its animals, such as a research institution, may use its own non-veterinary staff to treat its animals. Care must be taken not to allow lay staff to treat animals which, although part of a research programme, do not belong to the institution.

Difficulties may arise in the care of sick or injured free-living wild animals found by non-veterinarians. They may give emergency first aid but unless the animal is taken into captivity for further attention (in the case of protected species, in accordance with the Wildlife and Countryside Act 1981) then the restrictions of the Veterinary Surgeons Act 1966 must be observed. If the animal is in fact legally taken into captivity then the owner may, of course, treat it. If the owner seeks the services of a non-veterinarian, such as an animal shelter, ownership must be given to the shelter if it is to provide the necessary treatment. Brief and temporary restraint of a wild animal does not render it captive in the legal sense. Refer to *Rowley* v. *Murphy* (1964).

(b)   First aid measures taken by any person in an emergency to save life or relieve pain.

(c)   Anything except a laparotomy, done other than for reward, to an animal used in agriculture by its owner or a person employed or engaged in caring for such animals.

(d)   The castration of very young animals; the docking of a lamb's tail by a rubber ring within the first week of life. Debeaking, dubbing and desnooding by a person who is 18 years old (or 17 if participating in animal husbandry training under the direct personal supervision of a veterinary surgeon or at a recognised institution under the direct personal supervision of an appointed instructor).

Aspects of veterinary surgery which certain non-veterinarians may perform

(a) A person carrying out a regulated procedure under the 1986 Act.

(b) Doctors and dental surgeons carrying out treatment, tests and operations, and persons giving treatment by physiotherapy to an animal at the request of a veterinary surgeon. Doctors may remove organs and tissues from an animal for the treatment of human beings.

(c) Those authorised to take blood samples from farm animals and poultry under the Veterinary Surgery (Blood Sampling) Order 1983; (Amendment) Order 1988 No. 1090. The (Amendment) Order 1990 No. 2217 authorises the taking of blood from badgers

Similar statutory instruments have laid down provisions for the performance of various procedures on animals by non-veterinarians:

> Artificial Insemination of Cattle (Animal Health) (Amendment) (England) Regulations 2001 No. 380; 2002 No. 824; (Scotland) Amendment regulations 2002 No. 191; (Wales) 2003 No. 1131 (W. 118); (Northern Ireland) 2005 No. 264.
>
> Veterinary Surgery (Artificial Insemination of Mares) Order 2004 No. 1504.
>
> Veterinary Surgery (Rectal Ultrasound Scanning of Bovines) Order 2002 No. 2584.
>
> Veterinary Surgery (Testing for Tuberculosis in Bovines) Order 2005 No. 2015.

Details of the above statutory instruments and similar legislation can now easily be obtained online.

Non-veterinarians may carry out laboratory tests on material taken from animals by veterinary surgeons but care must be taken that any diagnosis or advice which is based on the results is given by a veterinary surgeon. It might be acceptable under the 1966 Act to state a treatment for a given condition as part of a discussion on remedies as long as no diagnosis is offered by the non-veterinarian.

Certain latitude is allowed as regards treatment of animals in agriculture but the involvement of a veterinary surgeon is always required in the following circumstances.

(a) A boar over six months must not only not be castrated without anaesthetic, but the operation must be carried out by a veterinary surgeon.

(b) De-beaking, by whomsoever carried out, must be performed as prescribed in the Veterinary Surgery (Exemptions) Order 1962.

(c) Dubbing (trimming of comb) of older birds should be done only on veterinary advice and by a skilled operator.

(d) Docking of the tails of pigs over seven days old is forbidden unless done by a veterinary surgeon on health grounds or to prevent injury from tail-biting (Welfare of Livestock (Docking of Pigs) Regulations 1974).

Special exceptions to the prohibition, contained in the Veterinary Surgeons Act 1966, on the veterinary treatment of animals by people other than veterinary surgeons were made for veterinary nurses in 2002. Veterinary nurses may do the things specified in paragraphs 6 and 7 of Schedule 3 to the Veterinary Surgeons Act 1966 (Schedule 3 Amendment) Order 2002 No. 1479. (consult RCVS Online > Veterinary Nurses at www.rcvs.org.uk).

Other persons with special exemptions are registered farriers in accordance with the Farriers (Registration) Acts 1975 and 1977 and physiotherapists, chiropractors and osteopaths in accordance with the Veterinary Surgery (Exemptions) Order 1962.

Treatment by acupuncture, aromatherapy, homeopathy or other complementary forms of therapy may only be administered by a veterinary surgeon, who should have undergone training in these procedures. Faith healers are required, in terms of the Code of Practice of the Confederation of Healing Organisations, to ensure that animals have been seen by a veterinary surgeon who is content for healing to be given by the laying on of hands.

Behavioural treatment that includes acts of veterinary surgery must be undertaken by a veterinary surgeon (cf. RCVS Veterinary Surgeons Guide to Professional Conduct: www.rcvs.org.uk).

If wildlife is temporarily caught for scientific purposes, such as to apply superficial monitoring devices or using painless methods of identification as long as no diagnosis, treatment or surgical intervention is involved, the activity is not governed by the 1966 Act. If veterinary procedures are involved they should be performed by a veterinary surgeon unless it is a matter of first aid or they are being performed as regulated procedures authorised under the A(SP)A.

A veterinary surgeon giving an anaesthetic in a regulated procedure must be authorised under the A(SP)A. The complex legal situation of veterinary surgeons operating as named veterinary surgeons or licensees under the A(SP)A has been discussed already in the Chapter 9. A letter in September 1998 from the Assistant Registrar and Head of Professional Conduct at the Royal College of Veterinary Surgeons drew attention to the intricate relationship between the A(SP)A and the Veterinary Surgeons Act 1966. A statement on the legal position of veterinary surgeons involved with both Acts accompanied this letter. In this statement issued by LAVA (British Laboratory Animal Veterinary Association) six principles of good practice in confronting conflicting legislative requirements were presented. These recommendations are relevant to veterinary surgeons involved with designated establishments.

Veterinary medicines

Since October 2005 new legislation has introduced drastic changes as regards drugs and medicines used by veterinary surgeons. The Veterinary Medicines Regulations 2005 No. 2745 provide a single comprehensive set of controls on all aspects of veterinary medicines other than residues. They replace in part the Medicines Act 1968 and approximately 45 statutory instruments that previously covered individual aspects of the production and placing on the market of veterinary medicines. These Regulations make provision for the authorisation, manufacture, classification, distribution and administration of veterinary medicinal products. They implement Directive 2001/82/EC as amended by Directive 2004/28/EC. Residues are not included because the European Commission is about to make proposals to revise the EC legislation [written in 2007]. These changes will be incorporated into the Regulations when they are agreed so that there will be a single instrument. The 2006 Regulations have advanced this process.

'Animal' in the 1966 Act

In the 1966 Act 'animal' includes birds and reptiles as well as mammals. Fish and invertebrates are excluded. Amphibians as such are not mentioned so in keeping with the dictum *Expressio unius, exclusio alterius* (what is expressed excludes others) it would appear amphibians do not come under the 1966 Act, at least until there is an authoritative decision to the contrary. Marine animals are within the scope of the Act.

Further changes after 2006

A further fundamental change is in the offing as regards veterinary surgery. A proposal to update legislation covering veterinary surgery was unveiled by DEFRA in September 2003. The associated consultation paper recognised that the Veterinary Surgeons Act 1966 was in need of modernisation and it invited comments on proposed changes.

Chapter 16

Drugs in Research

The salient pieces of legislation relevant to the use of drugs in research are:

- the Medicines Act 1968
- the Misuse of Drugs Act 1971

Many of the complex regulations associated with the two Acts referred to are outside the scope of this book. Most of the material, even regarding animals, is more relevant to a specialised work on veterinary medicine, particularly in regard to the 'cascade system'. This controls the dispensing practices of veterinary surgeons as regards the use, with the assent of the owner of the animal, of veterinary medicines not specific to the type of animal being treated, human medicines or a proprietary brand made up on a one-off basis. Since the main concern underlying these stipulations is in respect to possible hazards arising from pharmacologically active ingredients in the human food chain, it suffices, I think, merely to refer interested parties to the Medicines (Restrictions on the Administration of Veterinary Medicinal Products) Regulations 1994. These Regulations express in UK Law EC Directive 81/851 and the amendment to Directive 90/696. The Veterinary Medicines Directorate issued a clarification of these Regulations in a Guidance Note.

The Medicines Act 1968

The Act controls the sale and use of medicinal products – that is, any material given to a person or animal which it is expected will be of benefit to them. It also controls other substances and articles through a comprehensive system of licences and certificates, such as the Animal Test Certificate which permits the use of animals for the clinical testing of veterinary medicines without the need for either a Home Office Project or Personal Licence (A(SP)A s. 2(6) and the Medicines Act 1968 s. 32(6) and s. 35(8)(b)).

Misuse of Drugs Act 1971

The Misuse of Drugs Act 1971 lists and classifies controlled drugs and lays down restrictions on the importation, production, supply and possession of such drugs.

The Act provides strict and concise guidelines as to the storage of the drugs which it seeks to control the use of. In particular any room, cabinet or safe in which drugs are stored must only be accessible to a person licensed to handle or prescribe them. If controlled drugs are not so stored, the Act provides that 'as far as circumstances permit' they should be kept in a locked receptacle which can only be opened by authorised persons.

The Misuse of Drugs Regulations 1973, Part III, specifies the requirements for documentation and record-keeping. A record must be kept of drug use. Entries must be made in chronological sequence as set out in the Schedules. Each quantity of controlled drugs either obtained or supplied by a department must be entered in the register. A separate register or part of a register must be kept for entries of each class of drug and each of the individual drugs within that class, together with its salts. Any preparation or other product containing it or any of its salts must be treated as a separate class. Any stereoisomeric forms of a drug or its salts should be classed with that drug. These Regulations are frequently amended. For example, Misuse of Drugs (Amendment No. 3) Regulations 2006.

Registers

Regulation 19 sets out the following rules.

(1) The class of drugs to which the entries on each page of a register relate must be specified at the head of that page.
(2) Every entry in the register must be made on the day on which the drug is obtained or supplied.
(3) No amendment or deletion of an entry must be made. Corrections must be by a marginal note or footnote and specify the date on which the correction was made.
(4) Every entry and correction must be made in ink or other indelible material.
(5) The register must be used only for entries concerning drugs.
(6) Anyone required to keep a register must, on demand from the Secretary of State's inspectors, furnish particulars of drugs specified in Schedule 2 and obtained or supplied by him or in his possession. He must be able to produce proper documentation.
(7) Every register in which entries are currently being made should be kept at the premises to which it relates.
(8) All registers and books shall be kept for two years from the date on which the last entry is made.

Impact of medicine legislation on research

A person in charge of a laboratory the recognised activities of which include the conduct of scientific education or research and which is attached to a university or hospital maintained out of public funds or by a charity or other institution approved by the Home Secretary may possess or supply controlled drugs listed in Schedules 2 and 3 of the Regulations already referred to. Supply must be to a person legally entitled to have the drug in his possession.

Veterinary prescription–only medicines may be administered only by a veterinary surgeon or a person acting in accordance with the direction of a veterinary surgeon, whether they are required to be obtained on prescription from a pharmacy or through a veterinary surgeon or by a scientific establishment. The phrase 'in accordance with directions' has not been defined by the courts but it is considered that a veterinary surgeon has discretion as to what degree of direction, from verbal guidance to the actual overseeing of its use, he should give to a client. It must, however, be in accordance with the circumstances of the case because there may be the possibility of civil liability for negligent advice or supervision.

The controlled drugs most commonly administered to animals are contained in Schedules 2 and 3 of the Regulations. Those listed in Schedule 3, including barbiturates, are not subject to the requirements for record-keeping, nor is the strict standard set for the safe custody of other listed drugs demanded. These Schedules (which are liable to be added to or amended) can be obtained with a copy of the Misuse of Drugs Regulations 1973. Persons directly involved in these matters should consult this source material if they wish for clarification on the subject.

Under the Control of Substances Hazardous to Health Regulations (COSHH) 1994, medicines are only exempt from the relevant stipulations of the Regulations in the hands of the patient. Pharmacists, doctors and nurses are bound by the COSHH Regulations regarding the control and use of these medicines, and likewise veterinary surgeons and those in research institutes acting under their directions are similarly bound.

Poisonous substances which are not medicines are controlled by the Poisons Act 1972 and the Poisons Rules 1982 which restrict the supply of substances listed in the Poisons List Order 1978. Poisons must be sold through pharmacies except for Part II poisons which may be supplied by listed sellers to a person or institute concerned with education or research.

The significant implications of the Statutory Instrument, The Veterinary Medicines Regulations 2005 No. 2745, have already been stressed in Chapter 15.

Chapter 17

Liability in the Animal Unit

Liability in respect of the hazards arising from animals' aggressive behaviour, condition, or even presence is also a matter for consideration within the scope of animal law as well as the more discussed liability to animals in respect of the responsibility for their care. Most animal legislation, such as the A(SP)A and the 1911 Act, is of its nature concerned usually with offences involving cruelty or neglect, and so falls within the realm of criminal law. One piece of animal legislation, called simply the Animals Act 1971, does, however, belong within the range of civil law. This Act is mainly concerned with liability arising from the commission of various torts.

A tort, a civil wrong, is an unlawful act arising primarily from the operation of law. A tort gives rise to a civil action for unliquidated (a sum of money to be awarded by a court) damages, such as compensation to a person injured by an animal, or some other remedy; for example, an injunction may be issued in a *quia timet* (because one fears) action, where imminent danger is reasonably anticipated from the escape of a dangerous or infected animal. Such a mandatory injunction could impose strict conditions of containment. Non-compliance could result in the person responsible for the animal being held in contempt of court. In cases concerned with tort the defendant is sued by a claimant (previously known as a plaintiff); he is not prosecuted by the Crown. Redress is being sought for an injury through a decision from a judge adjudicating in a civil court. The Crown is present rather in the role of arbitrator than in the capacity of administering retributive justice, its prominent function in criminal courts. There is a significant distinction in civil cases as regards the burden of proof. The claimant is only required to establish his claim on 'a balance of probabilities' and not beyond 'reasonable doubt'.

A person may be liable for damage done by animals either in accordance with the Animals Act 1971 or on general principles in tort, for example strict liability, negligence, nuisance and trespass. There may be, in some cases, liability arising from a breach of a statutory duty. The legal action for injuries arising from these sources will be duly considered.

The Animals Act 1971

Following review by the Law Commission, the Animals Act came into force in 1971 and replaced the previously highly complex existing common law rules. One of the complexities of the common law had been the notion of 'scienter liability'. Animals had been considered in law as either *ferae naturae* (fierce by nature) or *mansuetae naturae* (tame by nature). The classification was a matter of law and was judicially noticed. In *McQuaker v. Goddard* (1940) it was judicially noted that a camel is a domestic animal and therefore *mansuetae naturae*.

Liability depended on knowledge (scienter) of the dangerous propensities of an animal by the one in charge of them. The owner of a *ferae naturae* animal was presumed to know it was dangerous. A claimant suing on account of injury from a *mansuetae naturae* animal had to prove 'scienter' – knowledge on the part of the owner that the animal was dangerous. Previous indication of a merely general vicious tendency of the wayward animal sufficed.

The new Act clarified this area of liability. It imposed strict liability (a topic which will be dealt with later) for damage done by dangerous animals. It defined dangerous animals as those species which are not commonly domesticated in the British Isles or those fully grown animals which normally have such characteristics that they are likely, unless restrained, to cause severe damage or that any damage they may cause is likely to be severe (s. 6(2)).

Where damage is caused by an animal which does not belong to a dangerous species the keeper is liable if:

'(a)   the damage is of a kind which the animal, unless restrained, was likely to cause or which, if caused by the animal, was likely to be severe, and

(b)   the likelihood of the damage or of its being severe was due to characteristics of the animal which are not normally found in animals of the same species or are not normally so found except at particular times or in particular circumstances: and

(c)   those characteristics were known to that keeper or were at any time known to a person who at that time had charge of the animal as that keeper's servant . . .'

(s. 2(2))

All this may seem far removed from research institutes, but not all laboratory animals are little mice well tucked away in cages. I have known a worrying experience of a frisky experimental goat escaping onto a suburban road just when nearby schools were closing and numerous drivers had hazardous close encounters with the creature.

In spite of the reform of the law, some features of the present legislation may seem a little strange.

'A keeper is not liable for damage caused by his animal kept on any premises to a person trespassing there, if it is proved either: –

(a)   that the animal was not kept there for the protection of person or property; or

(b)   (if the animal was kept there for the protection of persons or property) that keeping it there for that purpose was not unreasonable.'

(s. 5(3))

Liability of the staff of animal units

The Code of Practice of the A(SP)A draws attention to specific hazards associated with animals.

> 'Precautions should be taken in animal rooms to minimise the exposure of personnel to hazards which may arise from the incorrect handling of animals e.g. bites, scratches, allergens and infections and to prevent exposure to hazardous treatments intended for or applied to animals.'

This warning aptly applies to dangers in an animal unit from toxic substances, biological hazards and radiation. There are strict and detailed regulations covering the use of biological and radioactive material. This literature is referred to in the bibliography. It suffices here to mention COSHH 1994, particularly Regulation 10. Further guidance is given in *Surveillance of the People Exposed to Health Risks at Work* (Health and Safety Publication (HS(G) 61)).

The supply by the employer to the employee of necessary and appropriate personal protective equipment is mandatory under the Personal Protective Equipment at Work Regulations 1992 (SI 2966). These Regulations give effect to the Directive (89/656/EEC) on the minimum health and safety requirements with regard to the use by workers of personal protective equipment at work.

The Regulations require employers to:

- provide personal protective equipment (PPE) where risks to health and safety cannot be controlled adequately by other means
- select PPE that is suitable for the risks to be protected against (this could imply the need to provide protective gloves for the handling of primates)
- maintain PPE to acceptable standards and provide storage space
- ensure that the PPE provided is properly used
- ensure employees are given information on and instruction in the use of PPE supplied.

Monitoring of exposures and provision of health surveillance should continue, where appropriate, alongside the use of PPE.

Risk assessment

The likelihood of damage of any sort arising from dealing with the animals should be considered as part of the overall risk assessment of the animal facility. 'Risk' should not be confused with 'hazard' which is a potential danger, avoidable or unavoidable in certain circumstances. A 'risk' means that there is a reasonable probability of an unfavourable outcome. Risk assessment should contain an element of quantification, a probability measurement. Consequent on such an assessment there should be an agreed system of work and availability, if need be, of protective clothing as well as equipment and drugs for restraining purposes. Handling methods should balance minimum effective restraint and minimum risk. All those involved with animals must be trained in methods of handling and right use of methods of restraint. Licensee training in keeping with the Directive (86/609/EEC) and associated with the A(SP)A provides for this type of instruction.

In-house rules should be drawn up for dealing with large and dangerous animals. Particular attention should be given to the handling of infected animals as well as monkeys and venomous snakes. Any injury by an animal, however slight, must be reported immediately and appropriate action taken. Even the fluffy bunny can pack a good kick with resulting deep scratches.

> 'Where a person employed as a servant by a keeper of an animal incurs a risk incidental to his employment he shall not be treated as accepting it voluntarily.'
>
> Animal Act (s. 6(5))

This means that an employer cannot use a standard defence in tort cases, *volenti non fit injuria* – the claim that one who takes on a risk voluntarily cannot be injured in law. However, no one can be liable for injury to a person who is completely to blame for the injury he has suffered (s. 5(1)).

If injury to the plaintiff takes the form of nervous shock, such damage is actionable under s. 2(1). This section also gives grounds for claims for infection from a diseased animal.

Employees must take care of their own health and that of others with whom they are involved. They must not recklessly interfere with anything provided in the interest of health and safety (cf. Health and Safety at Work etc. Act s. 7). Supervisors need to be alert. Allowing a new young technician to go unattended among housed cattle would be irresponsible. Even experienced stockmen have been fatally injured in such circumstances (*Health and Safety Commission Newsletter*, October 1995, p. 10).

Zoonoses orders

The Agriculture (Miscellaneous Provisions) Act 1972 is concerned with the control of zoonoses. It is intended to reduce the risk to human health from any disease of, or organism carried in, animals. The Minister (within DEFRA) may by order designate any such disease or organism which in his or her opinion constitutes such a risk. There is a general directive providing the Minister with contingent powers to deal with special cases. For this reason the list of zoonotic diseases, transferable from animals to man, and recognised in law, needs to be and is constantly updated. The Zoonoses Order of 1975 exempted those involved in research from the requirement to report occurrences of brucellosis and salmonellosis (reportable diseases as distinct from notifiable diseases) in food animals. The Zoonoses Order of 1989 updated the list of dangerous organisms. Information of changes in the Schedule of the Zoonoses Order can be obtained from DEFRA.

The Code of Practice of the A(SP)A appropriately refers to this matter:

> 'Animals that may harbour zoonotic agents should be caged, managed and handled in such a way as to minimise any risk of infection being transmitted.'

COSHH assessment should take account of all possible zoonotic hazards resulting from the presence of micro-organisms hazardous to health. The consequences of the assessment should be strict control of contacts with possibly infected animals, prophylactic procedures where possible (e.g. vaccination) and strict adherence to quarantine rules. Regular checks must be available to endangered staff, for example for TB where staff are in contact with primates from the wild.

Industrial diseases

Some animal diseases are referred to in the Industrial Diseases Act 1981. Under the Social Security (Industrial Diseases) Prescribed Diseases Regulations 1985 (SI 967) there are prescribed occupational conditions or diseases which will qualify claimants to receive benefits. The list includes:

Anthrax
Avian chlamydiosis
Hydatidosis
Leptospirosis
Brucella infections
Streptococcus suis infection
Ovine chlamydiosis
Tuberculosis.

Amendments to this list, like the Social Security (Industrial Injuries) Prescribed Diseases) Amendment Regulations 2002 No. 1717, will continue to be issued from the appropriate department of Social Services. Text of such Statutory Instruments can be obtained at the website: www.opsi.gov.uk social security (industrial diseases).

Biological hazards

The Biological Agents Directive 90/679/EEC) defined 'biological agents' as micro-organisms including genetically modified organisms and cell cultures, and applies to work activities where employees may be exposed to such agents. The COSHH Regulations 1994 (SI 3247) and subsequent amendments thereof implement the European directives on the subject. The COSHH Regulations control the use of 'biological agents' in the workplace, and define more clearly the following terms:

> *Biological agent* – any micro-organism, cell culture, or human endoparasite, including any which have been genetically modified, which may cause any infection, allergy, toxicity or otherwise create a hazard to human health.
>
> *Micro-organism* – a microbiological entity, cellular or non-cellular, which is capable of replication or of transferring genetic material.

The classification and additions of newly recognised 'biological agents' is an ongoing process. The Amendment of the Classification of Biological Agents Directive (93/88/EEC) was discussed by the EC Technical Adaptation meeting (June 1997). Any proposed changes will duly appear in amended COSHH Regulations.

An abundance of Regulations have been issued as regards genetically modified organisms:

- Genetically Modified Organisms (Contained Use) Regulations 2000 No. 2831; (Amendment) Regulations 2005 No. 2466 and Regulations (Northern Ireland) 2001 No. 295.
- Genetically Modified Organisms (Deliberate Release) Regulations (Northern Ireland) 2003 No. 167 and No. 207; (Scotland) (Amendment) Regulations 2004 No. 439; (Wales) (Amendment) Regulations 2005 No. 1913 (W. 156); (Amendment) Regulations (Northern Ireland) 2005 No. 272.
- Genetically Modified Organisms (Traceability and Labelling) (Scotland) Regulations 2004 No. 438; (Wales) Regulations 2005 No. 1914; (W. 157); (Northern Ireland) 2005 No. 271.
- Genetically Modified Organisms (Transboundary Movement) (England) 2004 No. 2692; (Wales) Regulations 2005 No. 1912 (W. 155); Regulations (Northern Ireland) 2005 No. 209.

The text of UK Statutory Instruments can be found on www.opsi.gov.uk/stat.htm

For Scottish SIs go to www.opsi.gov.uk/legislation/scotland/s-stat.htm

For Welsh SIs go to www.opsi.gov.uk/legislation/wales/wsi

Northern Ireland Statutory Rules can be found at: www.opsi.gov.uk/legislation/northernireland/ni-srni.htm

Employer's duties regarding biological hazards

There must be an assessment of the risks of any work with biological agents likely to be hazardous to the health of employees. A distinction is made between workers who work directly with biological agents and workers where exposure may be incidental, for example maintenance staff.

Hazards may be prevented by substituting a non-pathogenic organism for a harmful one or treating organisms in such a way as to render them harmless. Control of exposure should be secured, where reasonably practicable, by means other than by personal protective equipment. The use of safety cabinets and isolators will sometimes be necessary. Specific guidance has been given in the *Code of Practice for the Prevention of Infection in Clinical Laboratories and Post-mortem Rooms*, issued by the

Department of Health. Four levels of laboratory containment are described corresponding to the four hazard groups. In future, of course, these may be added to or altered.

Employers are required to take all reasonable steps to ensure that control measures are complied with and that equipment is examined and maintained in an efficient state. Records of examination and tests must be kept for at least five years. Employees are required to make use of control measures and report any defects. (Health and Safety at Work Act (s. 7)).

Exposure of employees to biological hazards must be monitored. Records of monitoring of exposure of identified employees must be kept for *40* years. Health surveillance must be provided where:

(a) an identifiable disease may be related to exposure
(b) there is a reasonable likelihood that the disease will occur under conditions of work
(c) there are valid techniques for detecting disease.

The Reporting of Injuries, Diseases and Dangerous Occurrences Regulations 1995 (RIDDOR) require reports to be made to the Health and Safety Executive (HSE) of the death of any person as a result of exposure to biological hazards arising out of or connected with work and any potentially serious accident or incident, such as needle-stick injury where a pathogen is involved. There should be emergency plans for dealing with accidents with microbiological hazards. A code of practice has been issued by the Health and Safety Commission in connection with the COSHH Regulations 1994.

The Rabies Virus Order 1979 permits the importation, use and keeping of rabies virus only under licence.

All pathogens must be stored safely and securely with adequate labelling. Incineration, after autoclaving, is the preferred mode of disposal. Guidance from the HSE appears in *Safe working and the prevention of infection in clinical laboratories*.

Analogous regulations exist as regards exposure to radioactive hazards in the animal house. Naturally such regulations are stricter and vary as regards disposal of such hazardous material as isotopes. This subject is a very specialised area; it is not so relevant to most animal work. Council Directive (96/29/Euratom) revised the Basic Safety Standards Directive (80/836/Euratom) as amended by (84/467/Euratom). This new Directive was adopted in May 1996. Regulations based on this Directive can be found in publications by the HSE and on www.hse.gov.uk

Allergies

Laboratory Animal Allergy (LAA), a recognised clinical syndrome, can render a person unfit for work with animals. Since 1981 it has been a recognised industrial disease.

Occupational asthma from exposure to animals in laboratories was also recognised as an industrial disease in 1981. Cases of LAA requiring medical treatment and an absence from work must be reported to the HSE under the Reporting of Injuries, Diseases and Dangerous Occurrences Regulations 1995 (RIDDOR). The date of diagnosis, the nature of the disease and the occupation of the person affected should be recorded.

The COSHH Regulations 1994 require employers to assess risks of work with potential hazards such as animals, dust and disinfectants, control exposure, monitor control measures and provide health surveillance. This surveillance should identify symptoms of an allergy at an early stage. There must be provision of adequate ventilation and personal protective equipment, though the latter must be regarded as a second line of defence. As always, removal of the hazard, if possible, is preferable to provision of protection from it.

The whole topic of laboratory animal hazards has been comprehensibly dealt with in *Health and Safety in Laboratory Animal Facilities* (M. Wood and M. W. Smith, eds), a laboratory animal handbook (No. 13) published by the Royal Society of Medicine Press Ltd (1999).

Relevant torts

1 The rule in *Rylands* v. *Fletcher*

In *Rylands* v. *Fletcher* (Court of Exchequer Chamber 1866) Mr Justice Blackburn formulated the underlying principle: 'The person who for his own purposes brings on to his land and collects and keeps there anything likely to cause mischief if it escapes, must keep it in at his peril and if he does not do so, is prima facie answerable for all the damage which is the natural consequence of its escape.' This means that no negligence on the part of the defendant need be proved in a claim for damages caused on the land of the plaintiff which could be the expected result of the activity of an escaped animal.

A horsey story, albeit not very research-orientated, illustrates a possible association of animals with this rule. In *Jaundrill* v. *Gillett* (1996), a keeper of horses which had been maliciously released on to the road, where they panicked and galloped into an oncoming car, was not liable to a driver who collided with the horses. The Court of Appeal so held, allowing an appeal by the defendant against a decision in the County Court in favour of the plaintiff Jaundrill. Section 2 of the Animals Act (as presented in the early part of this chapter) was considered by the court.

The horses had escaped from a field where they were kept by Gillett. It was common ground. Some malicious intruder had opened a gate and driven the horses on to the highway. The only issue in the County Court had been whether the plaintiff was entitled to rely on what was basically the strict or absolute liability of the keeper of an animal other than a dangerous species. The plaintiff had relied on evidence of a veterinary surgeon that a group of horses when moved from their accustomed environment did tend to behave abnormally, and that horses removed from their field on to the road with other horses in the dark would tend to panic and gallop aimlessly in any direction. Mr Recorder Hussain in the County Court had found that the plaintiff had satisfied s. 2(2)(b) of the Animals Act. In the Court of Appeal, however, there were grave reservations as to whether a horse which galloped on a highway and panicked was displaying a characteristic under s. 2 of the Act.

Section 8 of the Act made express provision for the liability of a keeper whose animal escaped on to the highway through his own negligence. It was unnecessary to come to a conclusion under that aspect of the case. There had to be a causal link between the animal's characteristic under s. 2 of the Act and the damage done. In Lord Justice Russell's view, the real cause of the accident was the release of the animals on to the highway. Gillett's appeal was allowed and he was not liable for the damage.

2 Negligence

Negligence is the omission to do something which a reasonable man would do or doing something which a prudent and reasonable man would not do (Baron Alderson in *Blyth* v. *Birmingham Waterworks Co.* (1856)). Lord Atkin elaborated on this in *Donoghue* v. *Stevenson* (1932) (the case of the snail in the ginger-beer bottle): 'You must take reasonable care to avoid acts or omissions which you can reasonably foresee would be likely to injure your neighbour.'

Weller and Co. v. *Foot and Mouth Disease Research Institute* (1965) was a case where a research institute carried out experiments on their land concerning foot and mouth disease. They imported an African virus which escaped and infected cattle in the vicinity. Damages were paid to local farmers but in this case it was auctioneers who sued for loss of business because as a consequence of the calamity two cattle markets in the vicinity had to be closed. It was held by Mr Justice Widgery that as far as negligence was concerned the defendants owed no duty of care to the plaintiffs who were not cattle owners, and had no proprietary interest in anything which could be damaged by virus. Furthermore, the defendants owed no absolute duty to the plaintiffs under *Rylands* v. *Fletcher* (1866), because the plaintiffs had no interest in any land to which the virus could have escaped.

3 Nuisance

Perhaps this tort is less relevant to research establishments, though in the past debarking of experimental dogs had been considered so as not to incur liability for causing a nuisance to neighbours.

The tort of nuisance is based on the common law maxim *sic utere tuo ut alienum non laedas*: so use your own property so as not to injure your neighbour's. There have been numerous cases of nuisance involving animals as regards noise – cocks crowing (*Leeman* v. *Montague* (1936)), destruction of property by animals (*Farrer* v. *Nelson* (1885)) and smell (*Benjamin* v. *Storr* (1874)); Benjamin claimed that the smell from the excreta of Storr's horses outside his coffee house deterred customers.

4 Trespass

This tort is hardly likely to be of interest to research workers unless they are dealing with cattle. The Animals Act (s. 4) imposes strict liability for trespassing cattle, so no fault need be proved. The tort, however, is not actionable *per se* as it was in common law because consequent damage must be proved.

5 Breach of Statutory Duty

This tort is relevant to all the various COSHH Regulations referred to earlier and the following section on waste disposal.

To succeed in a claim in a case of breach of statutory duty the plaintiff must prove that:

(a)   the statute was breached
(b)   the breach caused the injury
(c)   the plaintiff was a person the statute was intended to protect
(d)   the injury was one the statute was intended to prevent.

A case which could be analogous to situations involving a duty to provide services such as adequate ventilation in animal units was *Bonnington Castings Ltd* v. *Wardlaw* (1956). The plaintiff was injured by inhaling silica dust because of the defendant's breach of the Factories Acts with respect to ventilation. Bonnington admitted the breach but denied it caused Wardlaw's injury. The House of Lords rejected this plea. Circumstances such as occurred in this case now come within the wider range covered by the Health and Safety at Work etc. Act 1974 and obligations are more clearly defined under the Workplace (Health, Safety and Welfare) Regulations stemming from the European Workplace Directive (89/654/EEC).

There was litigation concerning a university animal facility in which four technicians were awarded a total of £200,000 in out of court settlements after they developed asthma. Their complaint was that their asthma was due to working in inadequate ventilation (*The Times*, 21 November 1995).

Disposal of waste

The Code of Practice of the A(SP)A prescribes:

> 'A vermin-free collection area should be provided for waste, prior to its disposal Special arrangements should be made for handling carcasses and radio-active or other hazardous material . . . infected, toxic or radioactive carcasses must be disposed of so as not to present a hazard.'
>
> (2.33 and 4.17)

Animal house waste disposal may be subject to specific regulations and codes of such bodies as the Advisory Committee on Dangerous Pathogens and the Health

Services Advisory Committee. Animal carcasses from animal facilities are classified as 'clinical waste' in the Health Services Advisory Committee's guidance booklet. The safety policy should cover arrangements for colour-coding, segregation, storage, transportation and disposal of waste. Records of the disposal of radioactive material must be kept.

Local authorities may impose specific control on waste disposal. The Association of London Boroughs has issued 'Guidelines for the Segregation, Handling and Transport of Clinical Waste' (1989).

Non-domesticated animals

The Dangerous Wild Animals Act 1976, as amended, lists in a Schedule (which may vary in the future) non-domesticated animals which are considered capable of causing greater injury than a domesticated animal could. A licence is needed for the possession of these animals. Circuses, zoos, pet shops and designated establishments under the A(SP)A are exempt from the need to have a licence.

Chapter 18

Ecological Aspects of Animal Legislation

There is an abundance of legal material concerned with conservation. Most of such legislation is beyond the scope of this book. There is, however, some intrusion of this area of law into research. Ecologists holding project licences under the A(SP)A are not unknown, in my experience, either on remote Scottish isles or in wild areas of Wessex. Their targets of research are not within the confines of an animal unit. They may enjoy a free life closely associated with a PODE (place outside a designated establishment).

Categories of legal protection of non-domestic animals

There are several distinct categories of protection offered by the law.

(1) Conservation in general of wild animals. In law 'wild animal' is defined as any animal (other than a bird) which is or (before it was taken or killed) was living wild. (Wildlife and Countryside Act 1981, s. 27(1)). There is a presumption that an animal is a wild one, so the burden of proof falls on the person alleging captive breeding.
(2) Close season protection.
(3) Control of pests.
(4) Trade control. In this context 'sale' includes hire, barter, exchange and offering for sale. Restrictions imposed apply to parts of and products derived from the animal.

Much of our ecology legislation stems from International Conventions. They are the Bern Convention and the Washington Convention.

The Bern Convention

The Convention on the Conservation of European Wildlife and Natural Habitats (the Bern Convention) was adopted in Bern, Switzerland, in 1979, and came into force in 1982. The principal aims of the Convention are to ensure conservation and protection of all wild plant and animal species and their natural habitats (listed in Appendices I and II of the Convention), to increase co-operation between contracting parties, and to afford special protection to the most vulnerable or threatened species (including migratory species) (listed in Appendix 3). To this end the Convention imposes legal obligations on contracting parties, protecting over 500 wild plant species and more than 1000 wild animal species.

To implement the Bern Convention in Europe, the European Community adopted Council Directive 79/409/EEC on the Conservation of Wild Birds (the EC Birds Directive) in 1979, and Council Directive 92/43/EEC on the Conservation of Natural Habitats and of Wild Fauna and Flora (the EC Habitats Directive) in 1992.

The UK ratified the Bern Convention in 1982. The Convention was implemented in UK law by the Wildlife and Countryside Act 1981 (and as amended). As the inspiration for the EC Birds and Habitats Directives, the Convention had an influence on the Conservation (Natural Habitats etc.) Regulations (1994), and the Conservation (Natural Habitats etc.) Regulations (Northern Ireland) 1995, which were introduced to implement those parts of the Habitats Directive not already covered in national legislation.

The Wildlife and Countryside Act 1981 (WCA)

This is the main piece of legislation on conservation. It has been amended (1985 and 1991) and numerous statutory orders have been issued under it, such as the updating of Schedules which by their very nature require review.

The WCA makes it an offence:

- to take, kill or injure a wild animal (within the terms of this Act – those named in the Schedules)
- to have possession or control of, or to sell or advertise for sale, a live or dead wild animal (again within the terms of the WCA)
- to disturb, damage or destroy any structure or place used for the shelter or protection of wild animals (again within the terms of the WCA).

The WCA does protect birds in their own right. In s. 8, for example, it stipulates that birds can only be kept in cages of sufficient dimensions to enable birds to stretch their wings freely. Section 8 does not apply to a bird being examined by a veterinary surgeon, a bird being transported, or a bird being shown at exhibition, nor does it apply to poultry. It might seem that relief is given least where the shoe pinches most: Schedule 3, Parts I, II and III, of the WCA deals with the sale of wild birds.

The strictness with which the WCA is applied is illustrated by the fact that legal possession is deemed to arise independently of any intention on the part of the accused, thus creating an offence of strict liability.

Schedules of the WCA

The schedules of the WCA list the species of the animals protected (Table 18.1). However, conservation law is by no means static. For example, the 1985

Table 18.1   Schedules of the Wildlife and Countryside Act 1981 (WCA)

Schedule	Details
Sch. 1	Lists the birds protected by special penalties.
Sch. 2	Lists the species of birds which may be killed or taken outside close season.
Sch. 3	Lists birds which may be sold.
Sch. 4	Lists birds which must be registered and ringed if captured.
Sch. 5	Lists the species of animals which are protected. These include: some mammals some reptiles some amphibia some insects some spiders

Amendment of the WCA was repealed by the Wildlife and Countryside (Service of Notices) Act 1985.

In 1998, regulations added some species of animals to Schedule 5 and there were some deletions, e.g. the Carthusian snail and the chequered skipper butterfly. The WCA (Variation of Schedule) Order 1989/906 added 22 butterfly species. Examples of other Orders are those concerning coypus and seals. Obviously details such as these are only of interest to specialists in the field, but they illustrate the nature of the legislation.

Amendment of the WCA

There have been numerous amendments to the WCA. The 1991 Amendment, for example, varied permitted methods of killing. There have been changes to the species listed in the schedules, through variations to the Schedule's Orders. There is a statutory five-yearly review of Schedule 5 (Protected Wild Animals). This review is undertaken by the statutory conservation agencies and coordinated through JNCC (Joint Nature Conservation Committee). Changes to the Schedules can be made by the Secretary of State at any time, if it is considered necessary because of threat of extinction or in response to international obligations.

The Countryside and Rights of Way Act 2000 (CRoW Act 2000), which applies to England and Wales only, received Royal Assent on 30 November 2000, with the provisions it contains being brought into force in incremental steps over subsequent years. Schedule 9 of this Act strengthens wildlife enforcement. Schedule 12 creates a new offence of reckless disturbance, confers greater powers on police and wildlife inspectors for entering premises and obtaining wildlife tissue samples for DNA analysis, and enables heavier penalties on conviction of wildlife offences.

Other legislation relevant to ecology is Nature Conservation (Scotland) Act 2004, Local Government Act 1985, the Water Act 1989 and the Environmental Protection Act 1990.

The Conservation (Natural Habitats etc.) Regulations (Northern Ireland) 1995 is also relevant.

When citing any legislation, it is important to check whether any parts of it have been amended (or repealed) by later Acts or Statutory Instruments. Most UK legislation introduced since 1988 is available online from the website of the Office of Public Sector Information, http:www.opsi.gov.uk/legislation. If necessary, a qualified legal adviser should be consulted for definitive guidance.

CITES

The 'Washington' Convention on International Trade in Endangered Species of Wild Fauna and Flora, more commonly known as CITES, aims to protect certain plants and animals by regulating and monitoring their international trade to prevent it reaching unsustainable levels. The Convention entered into force in 1975, and the UK became a Party in 1976. The CITES Secretariat is administered by the United Nations Environment Programme. In 2004, there were 164 Contracting Parties and over 2500 species are included in the Appendices of CITES. Not all species are exotic; some are native to Europe and some native to the UK, for example the basking shark.

Species covered under CITES are listed in three Appendices, according to the level of protection they need.

Appendix I includes species that may be threatened with extinction and which are or may be affected by international trade. International trade in wild specimens of these species is subject to strict regulation and is normally only permitted in exceptional circumstances. Trade in artificially propagated or captive-bred specimens is allowed, subject to licence.

Appendix II includes species not considered to be under the same threat as those in Appendix I, but which may become so if trade is not regulated. International trade in these species is monitored through a licensing system to ensure that trade can be sustained without detriment to wild populations. Trade in wild, captive-bred and artificially propagated specimens is allowed, subject to permit.

Appendix III contains species that are not necessarily threatened on a global level, but that are protected within individual states where that state has sought the help of other CITES parties to control international trade in the species.

Each contracting party to the Convention designates a management authority which issues import and export permits for CITES-listed species based on advice from one or more scientific authorities.

The European application of CITES

CITES has been implemented throughout the European Union by EC Regulations. These impose stricter controls for many species than would be required by CITES itself.

In the European Union the CITES Appendices are replaced by Annexes to EC Regulation 338/97.

- *Annex A* – includes all species listed in Appendix I of CITES, plus certain other species included because they look the same or need a similar level of protection, or to secure the effective protection of rare taxa within the same genus.
- *Annex B* – includes all the remaining species listed in Appendix II of CITES, plus certain other species included on a 'lookalike' basis, or because the level of trade may not be compatible with the survival of the species or local populations, or because they pose an ecological threat to indigenous species.
- *Annex C* – includes all the remaining species listed in Appendix III of CITES.
- *Annex D* – includes those non-CITES species not listed in Annexes A and C which are imported into the Community in such numbers as to warrant monitoring.

The relevant regulations are:

Council Regulation 338/97 (Main Wildlife Trade Regulation) amended by 1497/2003, 834/2004 and 1332/2005 (amends all the Annexes)
Commission Regulation 1808/2001 (Implementing Regulation) came into force 19 September 2001.

These Regulations strengthen and extend previous import and export controls.

A principal requirement of these Regulations is the undertaking of checks on imports at the first point of entry into the EU, irrespective of the final destination. There are a number of areas where these Regulations are stricter than CITES, including:

- Some non-CITES listed species are included.
- Stricter import conditions apply for species in Annexes A and B.
- Import permits are required for all Annex B species and import notifications for Annex C and D species.
- Housing conditions are specified for live Annex A and B specimens (animals).
- Transport conditions apply to all live specimens (animals).
- More comprehensive restrictions are applicable for internal trade in, or commercial use of, Annex A specimens.
- Imports can be suspended of species that are considered to be an ecological threat in the European Community or of animals which have a high mortality rate during shipment or which survive poorly in captivity.

Users of animals in research need to be aware of the impact of EU Regulations on the movement and use of laboratory animals in practice.

EU regulation provides for the recognition of CITES licences issued by member countries. ESA (Endangered Species Act) animals taken from the wild within the EU and moved between EU countries require a certificate of origin. Specimens imported from outside the EU do not normally require additional permits on movements between member countries. There may, however, be specific national legislation on this matter which will need to be considered. Our own

UK law is liable to be more demanding in this area of importation of animals (cf. Chapter 22).

Council Regulation (EEC) 3626/82 on the implementation in the Community of the Convention on International Trade in Endangered Species of Wild Fauna and Flora required UK law to provide that endangered species must not be used for regulated procedures unless:

(1)   the animals are in conformity with the Regulations;
(2)   the research is aimed at the preservation of the species used; or
(3)   it is for a biomedical purpose, and the species is the only species suitable for the research involved (cf. Guidance 8.3, 6 and 7).

A general Index to EC Legislation can be found on the website of the European Commission which provides a search facility. More detailed information about the European Wildlife Trade Regulations can be found at www.eu-wildlifetrade.org. The European Commission have also produced a compilation report summarising points of interpretation and clarification of the EU Regulations.

CITES in the UK

The UK ratified CITES in August 1976. The Endangered Species (Import and Export) Act 1976 was the first piece of legislation to give effect to CITES. It has been substantially amended and is now largely superseded by the European Regulations. The Control of Trade in Endangered Species (Enforcement) Regulations 1997 (COTES) make provision for enforcement of the European Regulations. The Department for Environment, Food and Rural Affairs (DEFRA) is the CITES management authority for the UK.

As the UK CITES management authority, DEFRA is responsible for ensuring that the Convention is properly implemented in the UK, which includes enforcement and issuing permits and certificates for the import and export of, or commercial use of, CITES specimens. Applications for CITES permits are referred to a designated CITES scientific authority for advice on the conservation status of the species concerned.

JNCC

The Joint Nature Conservation Committee is the forum through which the three country conservation agencies – the Countryside Council for Wales, Natural England, and Scottish Natural Heritage – deliver their statutory responsibilities for Great Britain as a whole, and internationally. These responsibilities, known as special functions, contribute to sustaining and enriching biological diversity, enhancing geological features and sustaining natural systems.

As well as advising government on licence applications (*c.* 24,000 per annum) for CITES-listed species regulated under the European legislation, JNCC contributes to the development of government policy by providing sound scientific advice.

They also participate in delegations to national, European and international meetings, as well as assisting government with harmonisation of CITES procedures within the European Union and worldwide.

Specific Functions of JNCC are:

- to advise ministers on the development of policies for, or affecting, nature conservation in Great Britain and internationally
- to provide advice and knowledge to anyone on nature conservation issues affecting Great Britain and internationally
- to establish common standards throughout Great Britain for the monitoring of nature conservation and for research into nature conservation and the analysis of the results
- to commission or support research which the Committee deems relevant to the special functions.

For up-to-date information refer to www.jncc.gov.uk. Publications and checklists from the United Nations Environment Programme – World Conservation Monitoring Centre have been reproduced by JNCC (cf. www.jncc.gov.uk).

Enforcement of ecological legislation

Since 21/04/2005, COTES (Control of Trade in Endangered Species (Enforcement) Regulation 1997) includes new stronger powers of arrest, entry, search and seizure. Enforcement is the responsibility of HM Revenue & Customs and the police.

DEFRA's Wildlife Inspectorate works closely with the statutory authorities by:

- liaising and co-ordinating action with the Police and HM Revenue & Customs
- in the investigation and prosecution of wildlife crime
- co-chairing and providing a Secretariat for the Partnership for Action Against Wildlife Crime (PAW), a national multi-agency body looking at strategic enforcement issues and developing appropriate responses, in support of the enforcement of wildlife legislation
- managing a team of around 100 Wildlife Inspectors whose main role is to carry out visits to premises to verify information submitted for permits and certificates, or to check that people are complying with the administrative controls contained in certain wildlife legislation.

(cf. www.defra.gov.uk and www.ukcites.gov.uk and email cites.ukma@defra.gsi.uk.)

Chapter 19

Regulations Relevant to Animals in Research and the Impact of European Legislation

An open letter to Lord Sainsbury of Turville, the Minister of Science at the Department of Trade and Industry (12/06/2000) was sent by Professor Nancy Rothwell, MRC Professor of Physiology, University of Manchester and 109 other signatories, including five Nobel Laureates and 38 Fellows of the Royal Society, deploring the excessive amount of regulation and bureaucracy involved in the use of animals in research. It was strongly argued that the legal restrictions were seriously impeding the progress of research in the UK. This forceful document was concerned with the control exercised by the Home Office. The recommendations of the Report of the Expert Group on Efficient Regulation (October 2001), Chairman Professor I.F.H. Purchase OBE FRCPath, were directed at alleviating this grievance.

Unfortunately the Home Office is not the only source of regulations applicable to the use of animals in research. In the area of toxicology there is an abundance of regulations often of Byzantine complexity. Knowledge of their details and observance of their rules is vital to those working in regulatory toxicology. It would need volumes to do justice to this vast literature. Those involved in such investigation should consult the specific documents concerned with their work. The sources of testing regulations are the Regulatory Bodies, for example:

- National Institute for Health and Clinical Excellence (NICE)
- European Agency for the Evaluation of Medicinal Products
- UK Data Protection Commission
- UK Medicines and Healthcare Products Regulatory Agency
- UK Research Governance
- UK Health and Social Care
- US Food and Drug Administration

The Home Office published a Guidance on the Conduct of Regulatory Toxicology and Safety Evaluation Studies (2001).

US Food and Drug Administration Regulations

The USA Federal Register (Part II) is the source material for the FDA's GLP Regulations. These Regulations were instituted to assure quality and integrity of data submitted to non-clinical laboratory studies in support of applications to carry out clinical trials and the marketing of new drugs in the USA. They are, therefore, of great relevance to pharmaceutical companies involved in export of products to the USA. The sanction for observance of these GLP Regulations is the possible disqualification of the testing facility. Disqualification may be disclosed to the public. The FDA may inspect foreign (that is to the USA) facilities that seek a USA marketing permit.

Regulation of genetic manipulation

The EEC has issued Directives on the matter of genetic manipulation and, of course, will continue to do so. The principal instruments in this area have been Directive 90/219/EEC, On the Contained Use of Genetically Modified Organisms; and 90/220/EEC, On the Deliberate Release in the Environment of Genetically Altered Organisms (*Official Journal of the European Communities* No. L 117 8.5.90. pp. 1 and 15). These Directives have been translated into UK law.

The Health and Safety Executive (HSE) have published extensive information on this topic (cf. http://www.hse.gov.uk/biosafety/gmo/law.htm).

'The primary piece of legislation that applies to the use of genetically modified organisms in the workplace is the Genetically Modified Organisms (Contained Use) Regulations 2000 (GMO(CU)) and its amendment the Genetically Modified Organisms (Contained Use) (Amendment) Regulations 2002, and the Genetically Modified Organisms (Contained Use) (Amendment) Regulations 2005.

The GMO (CU) Regulations provide for human health and safety and environmental protection from genetically modified micro-organisms in contained use, and additionally the human health and safety from genetically modified plants and animals (GMOs). The key requirement of the GMO (CU) Regulations is to assess the risks of all activities and to make sure that any necessary controls are put in place. The GMO (CU) Regulations provide a framework for making these judgements, and place clear legal obligations on people who work with GMOs.

The Genetically Modified Organisms (Contained Use) Regulations 2000:

- require risk assessment of activities involving genetically modified micro-organisms (GMMs) and activities involving organisms other than micro-organisms. All activities must be assessed for risk to humans and those involving GMMs assessed for risk to the environment;
- introduce a classification system based on the risk of the activity independent of the purpose of the activity. The classification is based on the four levels of containment for microbial laboratories;
- require notification of all premises to HSE before they are used for genetic modification activities for the first time;

- require notification of individual activities of Class 2 (low risk) to Class 4 (high risk) to be notified to the Competent Authority (which HSE administers). Consents are issued for all Class 3 (medium risk) and Class 4 (high risk) activities. Class 1 (no or negligible risk) activities are non notifiable, although they are open to scrutiny by HSE's specialist inspectors who enforce the Regulations. Activities involving GM animals and plants which are more hazardous to humans than the parental non modified organisms also require notification;
- require fees payable for the notification of premises for first time use, class 2, 3 and 4 activities notifications, and notified activities involving GM animals and plants;
- require the maintenance of a public register of GM premises and certain activities.

There are also other pieces of health and safety legislation that are relevant to work with GMOs. These include the general requirements of the Health and Safety at Work etc. Act 1974, the Management of Health and Safety at Work Regulations 1999, and the Carriage of Dangerous Goods legislation. There are also some biological agents aspects of the Control of Substances Hazardous to Health Regulations 2002 which may be applicable in some circumstances. Further pieces of legislation covering the environmental risks posed by work in contained facilities with GM plants and animals are:

- Section 108 (1) of the Environment Protection Act 1990
- The Genetically Modified Organisms (Risk Assessment) (Records and Exemptions) Regulations 1996
- The Genetically Modified Organisms (Deliberate Release and Risk Assessment-Amendment) Regulations 1997

The Department for Environment, Food and Rural Affairs (DEFRA) is responsible for the regulation of deliberate releases of genetically modified organisms (GMOs). Further guidance can be obtained from the DEFRA website: www. defra.gov.uk.'

Other bodies besides DEFRA and the Food Standards Agency involved in the control of GMOs are:

- Department of Health – concerned with genetically modified organisms which have medical applications.
- Health and Safety Executive – responsible for compliance with regulations.
- Advisory Committee on Releases to the Environment (ACRE) – the statutory body which advises the Government on risks to the environment from the release of GMOs. ACRE carries out full risk assessments as regards GMOs and gives advice accordingly.
- Patent Office – regulates the patenting process.

Note: More details on control of genetic manipulation have been given in Chapter 17.

Good laboratory practice

Although somewhat on the periphery of legal control of animal use in research, good laboratory practice (GLP) is a very important issue in the pharmaceutical industry.

GLP embodies a set of principles that provides a framework within which laboratory studies are planned, performed, monitored, recorded, reported and archived. These studies are undertaken to generate data by which the hazards and risks to users, consumers and third parties, including the environment, can be assessed for pharmaceuticals, agrochemicals, cosmetics, food and feed additives and contaminants, novel foods and biocides. GLP helps assure regulatory bodies that the data submitted are a true reflection of the results obtained during the study and can therefore be relied upon when making risk/safety assessments.

The purpose of GLP is to control processes and conditions under which laboratory studies are planned, performed, monitored, recorded and reported. Adherence by laboratories to GLP ensures the proper planning of studies and the provision of adequate means to carry them out. GLP facilitates the proper conduct of studies, promotes their full and accurate reporting, and provides a means whereby the integrity of the studies can be verified. The application of GLP to studies assures the quality and integrity of the data generated and so qualifies for approval of the ensuing results by government regulatory bodies. Once approved by UK regulatory bodies such data may be accepted by foreign regulatory bodies. This is of special significance in hazard and risk assessments of chemicals.

UK GLP conforms with European Directives 87/18/EEC and 88/320/EEC. Even in a wider field UK GLP is in accordance with the standard set by the Organisation for Economic Co-operation and Development (OECD) (*GLP in the Testing of Chemicals, Final Report of the OECD, Expert Group on GLP 1982*).

Details of GLP

Details of GLP were presented in *Good Laboratory Practice: the United Kingdom Compliance Programme* published in 1989 by the Department of Health in London. Some details of GLP may be of special interest, particularly items of animal husbandry.

The application of GLP to the animal unit is concerned with:

(a) animal room preparation
(b) environment monitoring of animal rooms
(c) animal care
(d) handling of animals found moribund or dead on test
(e) identification of animals on test and correct allocation of cages
(f) cleaning of cages, racks and accessory equipment
(g) monitoring of food for analysis and shelf life
(h) monitoring of drinking water
(i) monitoring of bedding materials
(j) adequate documentation of all relevant observations.

Several developments have arisen out of GLP, notably SOPs (standard operating procedures). SOPs are written procedures which describe how routine operations, normally not specified in a study plan, are to be performed. The imposition of an extra condition on a certificate of designation is referred to in the APC Report 1997 (p. 24) and illustrates well the nature of SOPs.

'(xiv) That the applicant submits Standard Operating Procedures and protocols for the dog facilities relating to the housing, husbandry, care, restraint and performance of regulated procedures, with evidence that staff have successfully completed appropriate structured training. This should include:

(a) a protocol for the group-exercising of dogs which specifies that minimum daily exercise period per dog, defines the minimum amount of staff time to be used to socialise with the dogs, and identifies the type of area for the exercise to take place;

(b) protocols for the treatment of dogs to enable intravenous dosing and sampling and the proper production of haemostasis thereafter. Evidence should be supplied that animal care staff have been appropriately trained or re-trained.'

The legal status of GLP

The Medicines and Healthcare Products Regulatory Agency (MHRA) provide a comprehensive guide to UK GLP Regulations (cf. www.mhra.gov.uk).

'In 1981 the Organisation for Economic Co-operation and Development (OECD) principles of Good Laboratory Practice (GLP) were finalised and led to the OECD Council Decision: "Data generated in the testing of chemicals in an OECD member country in accordance with OECD Test Guidelines and OECD principles of Good Laboratory Practice shall be accepted in other member countries for purposes of assessment and other uses relating to the protection of man and the environment." At a meeting in 1983, concerning the mutual recognition of compliance with GLP, the OECD recommended that implementation of GLP compliance should be verified by laboratory inspections and study audits.

The European Community (EC) later adopted the OECD principles and a number of Directives stipulate that tests must be carried out to the principles of GLP and also that EC Member States must incorporate into their laws the requirement for all the non-clinical safety studies which are listed in the sectoral Directives, to be conducted to GLP and that premises conducting such studies must be inspected by a national authority. Consequently, on 1 April 1997 there came into force in the UK a Statutory Instrument (SI) entitled "The Good Laboratory Practice Regulations 1997" which superseded the voluntary United Kingdom Good Laboratory Practice Compliance programme. In 1998 the OECD issued the revised Principles of GLP and Compliance Monitoring. These were adopted by the EC in October 1998 and issued as Directives 99/11/EEC and 99/12/EEC. Consequently, in 1999, the UK Regulations were updated by SI 3106, as amended by SI 994, 2004, and are accompanied by a guide that interprets them and explains how compliance will be verified.

Responsibility for verification of adherence to the Principles of Good Laboratory Practice is a devolved matter, thus the UK GLP Monitoring Authority is a body consisting of the Secretary of State for Health, the National Assembly for Wales, the Scottish Ministers and the Department of Health and Social Services for Northern Ireland. Any one of the above acting alone or jointly may perform its functions. The UK GLP Monitoring Authority may appoint such persons as they think necessary for the proper discharge of their functions.

The Monitoring Authority formulates UK policy on the interpretation of the Principles of Good Laboratory Practice and responds to enquiries from industry, other Government Departments and other interested bodies in this regard. Biennial inspections of all laboratories within the UK that perform the regulatory studies that are required to be conducted to GLP are carried out by accredited inspectors. At present there are about 140 test facilities of all sizes in the programme. Other inspections verify the implementation of GLP for prospective members and surveillance inspections may also be carried out at the Authority's discretion.

The UK GLP Compliance Monitoring Programme is the mechanism whereby the GLP compliance of test facilities that conduct regulatory studies is assessed and monitored. In simple terms, test facilities are subject to routine inspections by the Good Laboratory Practice Monitoring Authority (GLPMA), the government body charged with enforcing the GLP Regulations. The GLPMA may also convene annually a meeting to provide a forum for discussions on all technical aspects of GLP.

Test facilities that conduct regulatory studies must, by law, be members of the Compliance Programme.'

Such regulatory studies are non–clinical experiments:

- in which an item is examined under laboratory conditions or in the environment in order to obtain data on its properties or its safety (or both) with respect to human health, animal health or the environment;
- the results of which are, or are intended, for submission to the appropriate regulatory authorities; and
- compliance with the principles of GLP is required in respect of that experiment or set of experiments by the appropriate regulatory authorities.

European legislation

The more important and relevant pieces of European legislation have been referred to throughout this work where appropriate. This seems to be the best approach to this intricate topic. We are not directly concerned with most of this legislation until it has gone through the UK legislative system either as an Act or secondary legislation such as regulations and orders.

The regulations of the kind referred to above result from European Directives which direct the governments of the member states to produce appropriate legislation on the matter covered by the Directive. Directives differ from European Regulations coming from Brussels in two important ways: they can be addressed to any one member state and do not have to be directed at all members of the EU; and they are binding as to the end to be achieved while leaving some choice as to form and method to the member state. Those Directives which apply to all member states have to be published in the *Official Journal of the European Union.*

Regulations coming directly from Europe are binding upon all member states and are regarded as directly applicable within all such states. Regulations have to be published in the *Official Journal* and come into force on the date specified in the Regulation.

Finally, decisions are commonly responses from the Commission to specific requests and are binding in their entirety on those to whom they are addressed. Our concern in the UK, therefore, is with European Directives which will eventually result in regulations from the UK government. Past Directives are already woven within this text.

A good illustration of how the process works is found in Directive 98/58/EEC concerning the protection of animals kept for farming purposes. The Council of Agriculture Ministers agreed a final text in June 1998 and the Directive was formally adopted in July 1998. This Directive sets minimum standards for welfare of livestock throughout the EU and a framework for adoption of more detailed standards for individual farm species. Article 3 requires that owners or keepers of any vertebrate animals kept for these purposes

> 'take all reasonable steps to ensure the welfare of animals under their care and to ensure that those animals are not caused any unnecessary suffering or injury'.

Any regulations issued on this material in the UK will cause little variation to our animal legislation. The terms of future regulations can hardly be predicted since Article 4 seems a little imprecise on the definition of 'animal'. We already have in place detailed regulations (the Welfare of Livestock Regulations 1994 as amended) stemming from the Agriculture (Miscellaneous Provisions) Act 1968 (cf. *Veterinary Record*, 14 August 1999, p. 178).

A further example of the influence of a European Directive on research is the 1993 version of the 1988 Directive on the patenting of biotechnology inventions. This new version stated that patents could not be granted on processes for modifying the genetic identity of animals which are likely to inflict suffering or physical handicaps without benefit to man or animal. The EPO (European Patent Office) granted a patent on the onco-mouse (carrying an implanted human oncogene) after initially rejecting it. In its final decision, it ruled that the benefit to humans of fighting cancer outweighed the suffering of the animal designed to develop cancer. This is an ideal example of official cost/benefit assessment. The decision opened the door to European patents on transgenic animals (LASA *Newsletter*, Spring 1993, and *New Scientist*, 16 January 1993).

The most significant piece of European Legislation affecting laboratory animals is the crucial Directive 86/609/EEC, frequently referred to in this text. It is specifically concerned with the protection of animals used for experimental or other scientific purposes. At the 19th meeting of National Competent Authorities on 29 November 2001, the European Commission announced that it intended to review and revise Directive 86/609/EEC. The Commission has set up a Technical Expert Working Group to assist in the review and revision of the Directive. The first meeting of the working group was held in Brussels on 30 June and 1 July 2003. The Chief Inspector of the Animals (Scientific Procedures) Inspectorate represents the Home Office on the Working Group. The eventual decisions of the Commission will probably initiate amendments to our domestic legislation.

Enforcement of European law

The Commission can refer cases of non-compliance with European legislation to the European Court. A complaint of the RSPCA was upheld by the EEC Commission which then referred the UK to the European Court for its failure to enforce, and in the case of France, for its failure to implement, the EEC Directive on animal transportation in 1977 and 1981.

The Council of Europe

The Council of Europe, based in Strasbourg, is a supernational body supported by agreement between national governments throughout Europe. Its influence is wider than that of the European Union, affecting states such as Switzerland, but it lacks direct legislative power. It considers the need to issue Conventions which serve as prototypes of relevant legislation in member countries (e.g. those in Table 19.1).

Table 19.1 Council of Europe Conventions on Protected Animals

Convention for the Protection of Animals during International Transport 1968
Convention for the Protection of Animals for Slaughter 1972
Convention for the Protection of Animals kept for Farming Purposes 1976
Convention for the Conservation of European Wildlife and Natural Habitats 1979
   (Berne Convention)
Convention for the Protection of Vertebrate Animals used for Experimental and other
   Scientific Purposes 1986
Convention for the Protection of Pet Animals 1987
Convention on International Animal Transport 1989

Table 19.2 Some international conventions on wildlife

Migratory Bird Treaties 1916–1976
International Convention for the Regulation on Whaling 1946
Convention on Fishing and Conservation of Living Resources of the High Seas 1958
Convention for the Conservation of the Vicuna 1969
Convention on Wetlands of International Importance especially as Waterfowl Habitat 1971
Convention for the Conservation of Antarctic Seals 1972
Convention on International Trade in Endangered Species of Wild Flora and
   Fauna (CITES) 1973
Convention for the Conservation of Migratory Species of Wild Animals 1979
Convention on Biological Diversity 1992

The UK's A(SP)A stems directly from the Convention which was adopted by the Council in May 1985, was opened for signatures in March 1986 and within two weeks had received the signatures of sufficient member states, including the UK, to bring it into force in October 1986, prior to ratifications by individual countries. As often happens with such Conventions, the EEC adopted a Directive (Council Directive 86/609/EEC) on the subject requiring member states to comply with the provisions of the Convention within three years. This gives the Convention legal bite on the European Union level. Further European Directives can be expected to be followed by UK regulations on material within the scope of this Convention. In January 1999 the first meeting was held in Strasbourg of the working party for the preparation of the fourth multilateral consultation of parties to the European Convention for the Protection of Animals used for Experimental and Other Scientific Purposes (1986). The text of the Convention ETS 123, Appendix A (on animal accommodation) was revised in 2006. The revision to take effect from 15 June 2007. Appropriate amendments will be duly expressed in our domestic legislation.

The boundaries of Europe no longer set the limits of the area which can influence our legislation. A parliamentary question to the President of the Board of Trade, asking if she would raise the issue of the effect of GATT on EU Animal Welfare Directives during the World Trade Organisation meeting in Geneva in May 1998, elicited the reply that the European Community's final position for the World Trade Organisation Ministerial Conference in May was still under internal EU discussion (*Hansard* 24/3/1998; Column 111).

The further broader legal dimension of international law is not usually of direct concern to the law-abiding citizen. In the area of animal legislation, one international convention is relevant in animal experimentation. The Convention on International Trade in Endangered Species of Wild Fauna and Flora 1973 (Washington Convention: CITES) was expressed in UK law as the Endangered Species (Import and Export) Act 1976. This matter has been referred to in Chapter 18.

Other examples, possibly of some interest, from the corpus of international law are shown in Table 19.2.

Chapter 20

Animal Welfare in Law

Animal welfare may be defined as the maintenance of animals under conditions of space, environment, nutrition, and so forth, consistent with the physiological and social needs of the species. This welfare is best achieved by good husbandry within the framework of the Five Freedoms.

Husbandry was defined by the Littlewood Committee (1965) as 'Routine application of sensible methods of animal care based on experience – a natural gift refined by study and improved by experience' (Littlewood Report, n. 201); in short, good stockmanship. An acceptable approach to animal welfare is ideally made through the practical expression of the Five Freedoms:

(1)   Freedom from thirst, hunger and malnutrition
(2)   Freedom from discomfort
(3)   Freedom from pain, injury and disease
(4)   Freedom to express normal behaviour
(5)   Freedom from fear and distress.

The concept of animal welfare is a relative latecomer to legislation. The Animal Health Act 1981 was a more positive approach to the care of animals than the previous basic Act in this area, the Diseases of Animals Act 1950. Even more positive was the further development, expressed in the title of the next Act, the Animal Health and Welfare Act 1984.

The early legislation on this topic was inspired usually by economic interests and so was concerned mostly with farm animals, with 'livestock' defined as animals kept for production of food, wool, skin or fur on agricultural land. The definition of 'livestock' applies to horses or dogs when being kept for the farming of land. Agricultural land is land used for the purpose of an agricultural trade or business. This legislation then is not applicable if the produce such as meat, milk or eggs are purely for private consumption (Agricultural (Miscellaneous Provisions) Act 1968). There are traces of earlier legislation concerning animal health than the Diseases of Animals Act 1950. Various pieces of legislation such as Statutory Orders were concerned with particular diseases, for example of cattle – Cattle Plague Order 1928. There was a long tradition of this type of ad hoc law making. An outbreak of disease among the cattle of Islington was met after, consultation with cow-doctors in 1714, by destruction and burning – by order.

By 1960 public concern was beginning to form about intensive farming and so there were motives, other than purely economic ones, to propose legislation concerning animals. The Brambell Committee (1965) examined the conditions in which livestock were kept and advised on standards of welfare. New legislation was the product of these deliberations. After the Farm Animal Welfare Advisory Committee (FAWAC) had been set up in 1967 the Agricultural (Miscellaneous Provisions) Act 1968 (A(MP)A) was passed to implement the findings of the Brambell Committee. This law made it an offence to cause or allow livestock on agricultural land to suffer unnecessary pain or distress. These terms were more clear and more embracing than the mere 'unnecessary suffering' of the Protection of Animals Act 1911. Detailed and practical Codes of Recommendation stemmed from the A(MP)A. The work of Professor Brambell continued and bore fruit in the formulation of the Five Freedoms in 1979 when the FAWAC became the Farm Animal Welfare Council (FAWC). The FAWC reviews the welfare of farm animals on agricultural land, at market, in transit and also at places of slaughter. The FAWC also advises the agricultural minister on any changes necessary to legislation.

Animal Health Act 1981 and Animal Health and Welfare Act 1984

The Animal Health Act 1981 was amended (particularly as regards animal breeding, medicines in foodstuffs and veterinary drugs) by the Animal Health and Welfare Act 1984.

Under this legislation MAFF (in 2001 DEFRA took over responsibility for this legislation) acted through the MAFF Veterinary Service (Animal Health Division) with enforcement by local authorities as regards:

- diseases designated as notifiable, e.g. anthrax and foot and mouth disease
- the eradication of such diseases as tuberculosis (hence the concern with badgers in 1999 in the West Country)
- the control of zoonoses and the institution of reportable diseases (zoonoses orders)
- the provision of a veterinary service
- the cleansing and disinfection of premises and vehicles (there are stipulations of great detail, e.g. types of disinfectants, under this heading)
- the slaughter and disposal of animals infected with notifiable diseases and compensation for their destruction
- the destruction of wildlife, e.g. in an outbreak of rabies
- the welfare of imported animals.

Disease orders

These were a major legal expression of the government's concern for animal health, such as the Pleuro-Pneumonia Order 1928 (Contagious bovine pleuro-pneumonia).

There is neither the space nor the need to deal in detail with the plethora of diseases orders in this book. In general the orders:

- limit outbreaks of disease
- promote the eradication of disease

by supervision of farms, markets and the movement of animals (often in great detail particularly in the case of pigs), and by supervision of animal importation. Most of these orders are extremely specific and may change frequently. They are usually only of interest to those directly involved, important though they are to those affected by them.

Up-to-date information on this legal material can be obtained from DEFRA. Suffice it here to refer to some significant ones to illustrate the pattern of this type of legislation.

The Psittacosis and Ornithosis Order 1953 introduced a category of scheduled diseases, such as chlamydiosis, as distinct from 'notifiable'. This Order was concerned not only with fowl but also birds such as parrots.

The Rabies (Importation of Dogs, Cats and Other Mammals) Order 1974 was within the enabling powers of the Diseases of Animals Act 1950. 'Animal' is defined to cover most warm-blooded animals – an animal (except man) belonging to the six orders of mammals in Schedule 1. Importation of such an animal is prohibited without a licence, a condition of which is isolation in quarantine for life if the animal is a vampire bat or for six months if it is an animal specified in Schedule 1, Part II (the effect of the European Belai Directive will be referred to later).

The Rabies Control Order 1974 was concerned with Schedule 1 of the 1974 Order. The Rabies Virus Order 1979 prohibited the importation of the lyssa virus of the family Rhabdoviridae (other than when contained in a medicinal product). The specific Rabies Act 1974 provided for the prevention and control of rabies.

The Zoonoses Order 1975 established a category of reportable disease. The duty to report is restricted to cattle, sheep, goats, pigs, rabbits, fowls, turkeys, geese, ducks, guinea-fowl, pheasants, partridges and quails (Art. 7). Outbreaks of salmonellosis and brucellosis in animals produced for human consumption must be reported to DEFRA which has powers to investigate an outbreak. Occurrences in other species need not be reported but DEFRA may investigate an outbreak which comes to its notice, for example through a veterinary investigation laboratory. There is no requirement to report the introduction of the disease into an animal for research purposes. Such animals must, of course, be disposed of without risk to human health. The Zoonoses Orders of 1988 and 1989 amended the 1975 Order and added to the list of dangerous organisms.

Medicines (Hormone Growth Promoters) (Prohibition of Use) Regulations were passed in 1988. Some exceptions were allowed under the European Communities Act 1972.

The Artificial Insemination (Cattle and Pigs) (Fees) Regulations 1989/390 are concerned with the need for official approval and an appropriate licence.

The Bovine Spongiform Encephalopathy (No. 2) Amendment Order 1990/1930 prohibits the use of specified offal in animal food.

These and other orders can be found in full with their amendments in Halsbury's Statutory Instruments and on the DEFRA website: www.defra.gov.uk.

Other disease legislation

A new and growing area of law covering animal disease has developed since the introduction of the Diseases of Fish Act 1983. The Act gave MAFF powers to deal with outbreaks of notifiable diseases in fish. It requires the registration of fish farms and stipulates that a licence from MAFF, now DEFRA, is needed for the importation of salmonid fish.

The Diseases of Fish (Definition of 'Infected') Order 1984 designated the following as notifiable diseases:

- bacterial kidney disease
- infectious pancreatic necrosis (IPN)
- viral haemorrhagic septicaemia (VHS or Egtved Disease)
- myxosoma cerebalis (whirling disease)
- infectious haematopoietic necrosis (IHN)
- ulcerative dermal necrosis (UDN)
- spring viremia of carp (SVC)
- furunculosis of salmon.

This Order applies to fish of any kind. Notification must be made to the Fisheries Department of DEFRA if it is suspected that fish at fish farms or elsewhere are infected with these diseases. DEFRA has powers to designate areas where there is an outbreak and to regulate the movement into and out of the area of live fish. The registration of inland and marine fish farms and shellfish farms carries the obligation to maintain appropriate records.

The Diseases of Fish Regulations 1984 define further the conditions on licences in respect to the provisions as to disposal, transport, inspection, cleaning and disinfection of fish or their eggs, their containers, the means of transport and any other conditions to prevent the spread of disease.

European legislative activity is developing in reference to infectious salmon anaemia.

There is a Bees Act 1980 which empowered MAFF, now DEFRA, to make provision for the control of disease in bees.

The above material is merely a taste of the complexities of the legislative attempt to control disease. I am sure it is enough for any reader apart from those with an avid interest in the topic.

The Animal Health Act 2002 supplemented existing powers under the Animal Health Act 1981 to facilitate the slaughter of animals to control the spread of foot and mouth disease. It provided for these new powers to be extended to other animal diseases by order. Additional powers were introduced to deal with transmissible spongiform encephalopathies in sheep. Amendments were made to the enforcement provisions of the Animal Health Act 1981.

Law and the killing of animals

Although the killing of animals is not *per se* illegal, this unfortunate procedure is hedged around by various laws prohibiting the killing of specific animals, such as the Protection of Badgers Act 1973; or concerned with the methods of killing, such as the Firearms Act 1968; or even the time of killing, such as the numerous and ancient Game Acts. The law may permit the killing of animals under licence, for example the Wildlife and Countryside Act 1981; or require the killing of animals, for example the Pests Act 1954.

This topic as regards laboratory animals has been covered in Chapter 5 under the heading of Schedule 1 of the A(SP)A.

The EU issued Directive 93/119/EC on the Protection of Animals at the time of Slaughter. This was implemented in the UK by the Welfare of Animals (Slaughter or Killing) Regulations 1995. These Regulations have been amended, so far, in 1999, 2000, 2001, 2003 and 2006. Guidelines were issued on the 2003 amendment. They dealt with licensing and training of slaughtermen, the alleviation of thermal stress in poultry in lairage and the slaughter of ostriches.

Significant details of these regulations are:

- It is an absolute offence to cause or permit an animal avoidable excitement, pain or suffering.
- There are specific rules on handling and stunning.
- Operators acting under these regulations must have the knowledge and skill to perform their duties humanely and efficiently.
- Slaughtermen must be competent and hold a Registered Licence.
- In every slaughterhouse there must be a competent person with authority to take action to safeguard animal welfare.
- Only permitted methods may be used to stun or kill animals.

Special methods of slaughter of animals permitted for religious reasons are confined to slaughterhouses. All licensed slaughterhouses are supervised by Official Veterinary Surgeons employed by the Meat Hygiene Service, part of the Food Standards Agency.

The Animal Welfare Act (AWA)

The best introduction to this crucial legislative venture governing the treatment of animals in England and Wales is to quote the Rt. Hon. Margaret Beckett MP, then Secretary of State for the Environment, Food and Rural Affairs, in the foreword to the Draft Animal Welfare Bill (AWB), July 2004.

> 'One of the frequent complaints made against the existing animal welfare legislation is that effective action cannot be taken where a non-farmed animal, although not currently suffering, is being kept in such a way that suffering will probably occur at some future point. This is clearly unacceptable and I

believe that a duty of care to promote the welfare of all animals kept by man is long overdue.

The creation of DEFRA in 2001 has brought all animal legislation – excluding that relating to animals used in scientific research – under one roof. This has provided a unique opportunity to embark on a root and branch modernisation of our animal welfare laws.'

It is obvious from the above that this new piece of legislation will not directly affect the legal control of animals used in research. The only part of the A(SP)A it repeals, is Schedule 3, paragraphs 1 and 7. These paragraphs merely refer to the references in the A(SP)A to two Acts: the 1911 Act and the Agriculture (Miscellaneous Provisions) Act.

Section 58 of AWA. (Scientific Research)

(1) Nothing in this Act applies to anything lawfully done under the Animals (Scientific Procedures) Act 1986 (c. 14).

(2) No power of entry, inspection or search conferred by or under this Act, except for any such power conferred by section 28, may be exercised in relation to a place which is –
(a) designated under section 6 of the Animals (Scientific Procedures) Act 1986 as a scientific procedure establishment, or
(b) designated under section 7 of that Act as a breeding establishment or as a supplying establishment.

(3) Section 9 does not apply in relation to an animal which –
(a) is being kept, at a place designated under section 6 of the Animals (Scientific Procedures) Act 1986 as a scientific procedure establishment, for use in regulated procedures,
(b) is being kept, at a place designated under section 7 of that Act as a breeding establishment, for use for breeding animals for use in regulated procedures,
(c) is being kept at such a place, having been bred there for use in regulated procedures, or
(d) is being kept, at a place designated under section 7 of that Act as a supplying establishment, for the purpose of being supplied for use elsewhere in regulated procedures.

(4) In subsection (3), "regulated procedure" has the same meaning as in the Animals (Scientific Procedures) Act 1986.

Attention has already been drawn, in Chapter 1, to the effect of the AWA on the 1911 Act and the 1954 and 1964 Anaesthetic Acts. The other animal legislation affected by the AWA is the Agricultural (Miscellaneous Provisions) Act 1968 (A(MP)A). The whole of Part 1 (ss. 1–8) which deals with welfare of livestock, codes, advice on welfare and the use of anaesthetics, is repealed by the AWA. The remaining parts of the A(MP)A deal with topics such as drainage, tenancies and miscellaneous provisions.

The DEFRA website provides ample information on this legislation. Those interested in the enactment and the details of the AWA should refer to: http://www.defra.gov.uk/animalh/welfare. The process of the legislation has been lengthy and complex. In clause 57(1) of the Draft it stated; 'This Act may be cited as the Animal Welfare Act 2004. Although on the DEFRA website we read: 'The 2nd Reading of the AWB in the House of Lords took place on 18/04/2006.'

According to the DEFRA website:

> 'The Animal Welfare Bill marks a milestone in animal welfare legislation. It brings together and modernises welfare legislation relating to farmed and non-farmed animals, some of which dates from 1911. Among other things, it introduces a duty on owners and keepers of all vertebrate animals – not just farmed animals – to ensure the welfare of animals in their care. It will mean that, where necessary, those responsible for the enforcement of welfare laws can take action if an owner is not taking all reasonable steps to ensure the welfare of their animal, even if it is not currently suffering.
>
> [. . .]
>
> It is hoped The Animal Welfare Bill will improve the welfare of all animals by tightening the legislation that protects them. There are three main areas which the Bill will tackle. Firstly, it will give welfare professionals greater powers to investigate incidents of cruelty and neglect. Secondly, it will enable action to be taken earlier to help animals kept in unsuitable conditions or without the care they need. Thirdly, it will increase the penalties faced by people who are found guilty of breaking animal welfare laws.'

The AWA will:

- reduce animal suffering by enabling preventive action to be taken before suffering occurs
- place on people who are responsible for domestic and companion animals a duty requiring them to do all that is reasonable to ensure the welfare of their animals
- extend the existing power to make secondary legislation to promote the welfare of farmed animals to non-farmed animals, bringing legislation for non-farmed animals in line with that for farmed animals
- simplify the legislation for enforcers and animal keepers by consolidating over 20 pieces of legislation into one
- extend to companion animals welfare codes agreed by Parliament, a mechanism currently used to provide guidance on welfare standards for farmed animals
- strengthen and amend current offences related to animal fighting
- increase the effectiveness of law enforcement for animal welfare offences
- increase from 12 to 16 the minimum age at which a child may buy an animal, and prohibit the giving of pets as prizes to unaccompanied children under the age of 16
- ban all mutilations of animals; however, there will be a regulation to exempt certain mutilations for which a ban is considered inappropriate – examples would be castrating and spaying cats and dogs, or ear-tagging cattle.

In defence of the Animal Welfare Act

DEFRA has issued various assurances on its website to allay the possible fears of stakeholders. A child will still be able to own a pet and a parent will still be able to buy a pet for a child under 16. Such a child, if accompanied by an adult, is allowed to win a pet. The AWA will not affect traditional field sport practices as free-ranging birds are considered to be wild and are therefore not protected under the Act. A Code of Practice will be produced to ensure that high welfare standards are met in the production of game birds for sport shooting. The welfare offence will apply to farmed game birds during the breeding and rearing process. The main provision of the AWA will not impose any new burden on responsible pet owners. The majority of animal owners already ensure the welfare of their animals and will not be affected by the enactment. The Act will, however, enable enforcement agencies to deal more effectively with the minority who fail to apply good standards. Anything which occurs in the normal course of fishing is exempted entirely from the Act. However, all fish for which a person is responsible are protected by both the cruelty offence and the duty to ensure welfare.

The purpose of this Act is to bring legislation concerning the welfare of other animals into line with that for farmed animals and consolidate it in one place. It does not constitute a major change for farmers.

Significant legal details of the Animal Welfare Act

Definitions of 'animal' within the context of the AWA.

'(1)   Subject to the provisions of this section, in this Act "animal" means a vertebrate other than man.

(2)   Nothing in this Act applies to an animal while it is in its foetal, larval or embryonic form.

(3)   The appropriate national authority may by order for all or any of the purposes of this Act –
   (a)   extend the definition of "animal" so as to include invertebrates of any description;
   (b)   make provision in lieu of subsection (2) as respects any invertebrate so included;
   (c)   amend subsection (2) to extend the application of this Act to an animal from such earlier stage of its development as may be specified in the order.

(4)   No order under subsection (3) may be made by the Secretary of State unless a draft of the instrument containing the order has been laid before and approved by a resolution of each House of Parliament.

(5)   In this section, "vertebrate" means any animal of the Sub-phylum Vertebrata of the Phylum Chordata and "invertebrate" means any animal not of that Sub-phylum.'

The explanatory notes of the Draft enlarged upon the legal text.

'200. This clause specifies the categories of animal to which the Act applies. The Bill affords protection to vertebrate animals other than man. The restriction to vertebrates is made on the basis that there is insufficient evidence to show conclusively that invertebrates are capable of experiencing pain, suffering and distress. There is an order making power to extend the definition to invertebrates or to particular types of invertebrates. This power would be exercised if scientific evidence demonstrated in future that such animals can in fact experience pain, suffering and distress.

201. Subsection (1) provides the definition of animal.

202. Subsection (2) specifies that the Act does not apply to unborn animals.

203. Subsection (3) sets out the ways in which the power to extend the definition of animal may be exercised. This includes a power to extend protection to unborn animals.

204. Subsection (4) provides for an affirmative parliamentary procedure in respect of the order making power in subsection (3).

205. Subsection (5) provides definitions of vertebrate and invertebrate.'

The enabling process will apply to this legislation. The DEFRA website explained this aspect of the Bill.

'The AWB sets out a broad framework and leaves much of the detail to secondary legislation that can be amended and revised more easily should the need arise. To a large extent the power to make secondary legislation replicates existing powers for farmed animals and simply extends it to non-farmed animals. The Bill also brings current licensing powers into one place. The Bill therefore provides an entirely reasonable level of regulation-making power. Detailed legislation on specific sectors or practices, including bans if appropriate, will be addressed by secondary legislation. This way it can be changed relatively easily in accordance with changing science and the values of society. There will be public consultation and the opportunity for everyone to comment before an area is regulated in such a way.
[. . .]
The Government is currently considering the case for using these powers to introduce some form of regulation for those who train animals to perform.'
(DEFRA website, November 2005)

The DEFRA website explained clearly how this legislation is to be enforced.

'Enforcement of the provisions of the Bill will be carried out by the police, Local Authorities and the State Veterinary Service, who will be able to recruit the assistance of other specialists such as veterinary surgeons where appropriate. We anticipate that most of the day-to-day enforcement work relating to farm animals will continue to be undertaken by the State Veterinary Service.'

'Local Authorities will also be able to appoint inspectors who are considered suitable for appointment on a temporary basis, e.g. a British Horse Society Inspector helping out in an area where there is a particularly high concentration of livery yards and riding schools. However, LAs will not appoint an organisation en masse to carry out LA functions. In particular, concerns that the RSPCA may be appointed en masse as local authority inspectors are misplaced. The appointment of inspectors will be based on the expertise of the individual concerned.'

'We anticipate that most of the day-to-day enforcement work relating to pet animals will continue to be undertaken by the RSPCA, who have undertaken the majority of cruelty prosecutions in the past under the 1911 Act. We anticipate that the RSPCA will also undertake the majority of prosecutions under the new welfare offence, though the RSPCA estimate that this will only lead to an additional 100 or so prosecutions a year.'

'However, as now, where access to premises is sought, the RSPCA will have to be accompanied by a Local Authority inspector or constable who has powers of entry under the Bill.'

'The RSPCA has long established expertise in both the investigation and prosecution of cases involving animal welfare. Animal welfare law has been common enforcer's law – anyone is entitled to bring a prosecution – since Parliament began legislating on it. To take away the power of the RSPCA to bring prosecutions would not only put an unreasonable enforcement burden on the police, but would be to the detriment of animal welfare.'

The AWA will apply to the Crown and so will bind all government departments and other public bodies. It only applies to England and Wales; similar legislation will be enacted in Scotland. The Scottish Animal Health and Welfare Act reflects the agreed consensus on the best way to solve problems which have been identified in Scotland, England and Wales. There are some differences which arise, in some cases, simply from different drafting preferences and, in some cases, from the different priorities of the two governments. The Scottish legislation is the Animal Health and Welfare (Scotland) Act. Statutory Instrument 3407 Animal Health and Welfare (Scotland) Act 2006. (Consequential Provisions) (England and Wales) Order 2006 is associated with the Scottish Act.

Chapter 21

Legal Aspects of the Transport of Animals

Correct transport of animals is an important feature of animal welfare. Many laboratory animals may never leave the animal unit where they were born, and even if they do, the time spent in transport will be a very small fragment of their total life. Nevertheless, such transportation may prove to be the most traumatic experience of their whole life, particularly at times of loading and unloading. The legislation concerning the transit of animals is perhaps the most complex, extensive and detailed area of animal law, especially as regards pigs. The difficulty here has been trying to avoid referring to endless minutiae. Such fascinating detail as the permitted method of sending leeches by post would no doubt be of great importance to some specialists but of little interest to most technicians, scientists or farmers working with animals.

The development of the law on the transport of animals

There have been numerous transit orders regarding animals in the past, such as the Transit of Animals Order 1927. Some referred to particular species of animals, for example the Conveyance of Live Poultry Order 1919, or were concerned with specific forms of transport – the Transport of Animals (Road and Rail) Order 1975. The Transit of Animals (General) Order 1973 was a milestone in animal transport law. Such orders as the Transport of Animals (Cleaning and Disinfection) Order 1999 (implementing European Directives 91/628/EEC, 92/65/EEC, and 97/12/EC on cleansing and disinfection in animal transport) will continue to be issued in the future. The most comprehensive piece of animal transport legislation has been the Welfare of Animals (Transport) Order 1997 (WATO), of which more later. It is the responsibility of those involved in moving animals around to keep abreast of developing legislation through contact with DEFRA, though future legislation in this area will stem from Council Regulation (EC) No. 1/2005. The DEFRA website is at www.defra.gov.uk

Apart from legislation there are other rules governing the correct transport of animals. The International Air Transport Association (IATA) issue annually the standards of packaging and so on which they demand before they will accept animals for air transport. The 32nd edition of these regulations was issued on 12 November 2005. These stipulations are mandatory on member airlines. MAFF produced a code of practice for the air carriage of farm animals and recommended conditions applicable particularly to endangered species. The railways have regulations regarding the carriage of animals. In literature issued on this matter, the need to care for all animals in transit was emphasised with the slogan 'Animals can't complain'. So solicitous was British Rail for animal travellers that it would not transport mice on high-speed trains, being aware of the deleterious effect on mice of excessive noise or vibration. The Post Office stipulates its own requirements on the mailing of invertebrates.

The various transit orders may have been detailed, but in the context of law they have been relatively clear. In practice, however, some cases resulting from this form of legislation may seem a little bewildering to the layperson. *British Airways Board* v. *Wiggins* (1977) involved two crates of tortoises transported from Amsterdam to Heathrow. Although British Airways staff did not load the crates, it was held that the airline was guilty of an offence under the Transit of Animals (General) Order 1973. The magistrates decided that even from a glimpse at the crates it should have been obvious that the receptacles were unsuitable. The tortoises were stacked in columns of six, one on top the other. In some cases their bodies were protruding through the slats in the side of the boxes.

British Airways appealed on the grounds that the offence was committed outside UK jurisdiction. The Lord Chief Justice, Lord Widgery, dismissed the appeal in the Divisional Court. There had been a continuing duty on the carrier to ensure that the containers would be adequate. The offence was committed on landing just as much as on taking off.

This case established that the carrier or any other person having charge of an animal is responsible throughout its journey for the provision of a suitable receptacle for it.

The House of Lords decided in *Air India* v. *Wiggins* (1980) that a carrier would be in breach of the Transit of Animals (General) Order 1973 if it carried animals in unsuitable containers or in conditions which caused unnecessary suffering when entering British territory. The carrier could be prosecuted even if it was not based in the UK and even if the journey commenced abroad. Air India, however, won its appeal against conviction. On appeal, Lord Scarman decided that no crime had been committed in the UK against the 2031 dead parakeets out of the 2120 parakeets transported from India to Heathrow. Engine trouble had delayed the aircraft for 31 hours in Kuwait. The 2031 dead birds had never been landed in the UK, only their carcasses. The charge in respect to the 89 living birds which had been landed and had also been exposed to the gruelling journey with insufficient ventilation was also quashed at the appeal. The legal reason for the dismissal of this part of the prosecution was that it was impossible to identify which crates contained the live birds. It seems Air India had no liability for a cargo of unidentified live birds nor for birds already deceased outside the UK.

The movement of laboratory animals

The Code of Practice for the Housing and Care of Animals used in Scientific Procedures has a section on this topic on p. 13:

'3.11   Stress during transport should be minimised by making animals as comfortable as possible in their containers and, if confinement is to be prolonged, by providing food and water. Time in transit should be kept to a minimum. Animals that are incompatible should not be transported together.

3.12 The sender should ensure that the animals to be transported are in good health and that their containers are adequately labelled. Sick or injured animals should be transported only for purposes of treatment, diagnosis or emergency slaughter.

3.13 Pregnant animals need special care. Farm animals should not normally be transported during the last week of pregnancy and small animals in the last fifth of pregnancy.

3.14 Where animals are subject to control under the Act, it is necessary to consult the Inspector about authority to transfer them to other designated premises.'

There is a special application form for authority to transfer protected animals. The form must be used if authority is not already incorporated into the project licence(s) or conditions on licence(s) or Certificates. This form can be found on the Home Office website: http://scienceandresearch.homeoffice.gov.uk/.

Besides the usual information and assurances sought on applications of this nature, the following notes are of special significance:

- 'If transfer might have significant health or welfare problems for the animals, indicate what these problems might be and what steps will be taken to minimise such problems during transport and on receipt.
- The reason justifying the transfer of the animals must be indicated on the application form.
- There must be a guarantee that the transfer will be in keeping with all relevant regulations regarding welfare of animals in transit and the legal requirements for the import/export of animals.
- The animals must be inspected by a competent person before and after transfer.
- Any necessary veterinary certification must be provided.
- Any welfare problem arising as a consequence of the transfer will be notified to the Home Office promptly.
- In all cases where the animals are not solely under a Certificate of Designation the appropriate PL holder [*sic*] is responsible for the animals while they are alive within UK jurisdiction.'

The APC has displayed a keen interest in the welfare of laboratory animals during transport. The APC (1998) Report published a pertinent and topical news item on the transport of laboratory animals:

'34. During 1998, the Animal Procedures Committee was extremely concerned to learn of the deaths of three primates in transit to the UK. The Home Office took immediate action, suspending authority to acquire animals from the source involved while the causes were investigated. Later, it emerged that it had not been possible to ascertain the causes of death. But it is likely that they were due to a combination of factors:

(i)   the animals concerned were larger than normal;

(ii)   although International Air Transport Association minimum dimensions were not breached, the containers were not large enough for these particular animals – they did not allow the animals to stand up and turn around freely; and

(iii) all the dead animals had been in central compartments, which were less well ventilated.

35. The Committee understands that the breeding establishment co-operated fully and immediately redesigned the containers to improve ventilation and to increase their size, and that the Home Office has now renewed authority to acquire animals from this source, subject to there being no further problems.'

(p. 7)

In the APC Report of the Cost/Benefit Working Group (17/06/03) attention was drawn to the 'cost' involved in the transport of protected animals (p. 83, No. 6.5.2).

'costs due to transport of all species covered by the Act should be included in cost/benefit assessments under the Act. Currently, only the adverse effects of transport of non-human primates are required to be considered as part of the assessment of costs, yet prolonged transport is also a problem for other animals such as genetically modified mice which have often been developed in and therefore must be transported from mainland Europe or the United States, or even further afield.'

Further material on this topic can be found in a valuable article in *Laboratory Animals* (2005) 39: 139, titled 'Guidance on Transport of Laboratory Animals'. It is a thorough report that accomplishes its goal of rewriting the existing UK Guidelines on the transport of laboratory animals, first published in 1992. The Working Group consisted of UK leaders in the fields of animal transportation and laboratory care from industry, academia and the private sector and was chaired by Jeremy Swallow of Pfizer.

Council Regulation (EC) No. 1/2005 on the Protection of Animals During Transport and Related Operations

From 5 January 2007, a new Regulation on the protection of animals during transport will apply across the European Union (EU), with some elements coming into force later in 2008 or in 2009. It will replace European Directive 91/628. The Welfare of Animals (Transport) Order 1997 (WATO) and its equivalent in Northern Ireland, which implemented the Directive, will accordingly be replaced with new Orders in England, Scotland, Wales and Northern Ireland. These will put the arrangements for complying with the new EU Regulation in place.

This fundamental change to our well-established animal legislation is one of legal principle rather than welfare content. The broad outline of WATO will be retained in practice, which made it an offence to transport any animal:

- in any way that is likely to cause injury or unnecessary suffering
- that is unfit to be transported
- unless there are arrangements for its care, both during the journey and at its destination
- by using excessive force to control it – the use of sticks, whips, crops and goads are also restricted.

We are, however, in the midst of an ongoing law-making process. Any inclusion of defined details of European legislation would not only be inappropriate in this text but could prove misleading. Part of the ongoing process has been a consultation exercise on the Implementation of EU Regulation 1/2005 issued by DEFRA. A deadline for comments was 31/07/2006. Up-to-date information on the progress of this legislation can be obtained on the website of the European Commission at: http://europa.eu.int/eur-lex/lex/LexUriServ/site/en/oj/2005/l003/1003200501053n00010044.pdf

The Regulation will apply to all those involved with the transport of vertebrate animals in connection with an economic activity; for example, livestock and equine hauliers, farmers, animal breeders, performing animal transporters and those working at markets, assembly centres and slaughterhouses. It would not apply to individuals who ride for pleasure and who transport their own horses, or to individuals taking their own pets on holiday. On the Home Office's application form for the transfer of animals under A(SP)A, it is a requirement that the applicant observe all relevant animal transport regulations. It will be incumbent therefore on those who transport protected animals to be attentive to this Regulation.

The Regulation amounts to a radical overhaul of the existing EU rules on animal transport and it identifies the chain of all those involved in animal transport, defining 'who is responsible for what' and thus facilitating more effective enforcement of the new rules.

The Regulation applies to the commercial transport of all vertebrate animals. Some requirements apply only to horses, farmed animals (cattle, sheep, goats and pigs) and poultry.

Although it has already been pointed out that it would be in vain, at this juncture, to attempt to spell out in detail the full impact of Regulation (EC) No. 1/2005, some indication of the main provisions of the new legislation would not be out of place. These provisions arise from the stated fundamental principle:

> 'No animal shall be transported unless it is fit for the intended journey, and all animals shall be transported in conditions guaranteed not to cause them injury or unnecessary suffering.'

Table 21.1   Requirements for food, water and rest

Species	First leg of journey	Mid journey rest	Final leg of journey
Unweaned calves, lambs, kids and foals which are still on a milk diet and unweaned piglets	A maximum of 9 hours	At least one hour	Then a further maximum of 9 hours
Other cattle, sheep and goats	A maximum of 14 hours	At least one hour	Then a further maximum of 14 hours
Pigs other than unweaned piglets	A maximum of 24 hours with continuous access to liquid		
Horses other than unweaned foals (excluding registered horses)	A maximum of 24 hours with liquid and, if necessary, food every 8 hours		

There are provisions relating to bedding, food, water, ventilation, access to the animals and the correct partitioning of animals.

Maximum journey times for farm animals and horses (including feeding, watering and rest periods) are linked to vehicle standards. Requirements for food, water and rest are shown in Table 21.1. These requirements may be amended in 2007 or after.

After the maximum permitted journey time the animals must be unloaded from the vehicle, fed, watered and rested for a minimum of 24 hours. This must be at an EU Approved Staging Point.

Unless exempt, transporters of animals carrying out journeys of up to eight hours will have to:

- be authorised by the competent authority (the authorisation will be valid for five years)
- have received training and (if transporting horses, farmed animals or poultry) have independent certification of competence approved by the competent authority
- demonstrate that they have appropriate staff and equipment to transport animals in a proper way and have no record of serious infringements of animal welfare legislation in the preceding five years.

Transporters carrying out journeys of over eight hours by road have to have their vehicles or livestock containers inspected and approved according to specific criteria. These will provide for:

- on-vehicle drinking systems
- ventilation systems capable of ensuring even distribution of air and being operated for at least four hours independently of the vehicle engine

- temperature monitoring and recording and a system to alert the driver to potential problems.

In addition, from 2007 new vehicles – and from 2009 all vehicles – used to transport horses or farmed animals on journeys of over eight hours by road will have to be equipped with a satellite navigation system to trace and verify compliance with travel limits for animals.

Unfit animals are more tightly defined and there will be a ban on transporting very young animals except if the journey is less than 100 km. For example:

- calves of less than ten days of age
- pigs of less than three weeks
- lambs of less than one week.

Exemptions are allowed for under the Regulation, for example:

- Journeys to or from a veterinary practice or clinic under the advice of a veterinarian are exempted.
- Farmers transporting their own animals in their own vehicles under 50 km are exempted from requirements for authorisation, training and certificates of competence.
- Transporters of animals for up to 65 km are exempted from requirements for authorisation, training and certificates of competence.

In the last two exemptions general conditions must be complied with, such as

- ensuring the journey time is kept to a minimum, and the animals are checked and their needs met during the journey
- the animals are fit to travel
- the vehicle and loading and unloading facilities are designed, constructed and maintained to avoid injury and suffering
- those handling animals are trained or competent in the task and do not use violence or any methods likely to cause unnecessary fear, injury or suffering
- water, feed and rest are given to the animals as needed; and sufficient floor space and height is allowed.

The introduction of new rules under Regulation (EC) No. 1/2005 has already been proposed, for example:

- From 5 January 2008, drivers and attendants on journeys of over 65 km must hold a certificate of competence if transporting horses, cattle, sheep, goats, pigs or poultry.
- Satellite navigation systems will become obligatory in road vehicles transporting livestock for over eight hours. For newly built vehicles it will become obligatory from January 2007, and for all vehicles from January 2009.
- There will be further proposals on journey times, resting periods and space allowances which are required to be reviewed by 2011.

This Regulation should improve animal welfare in transport throughout the European Union. Exchange of information between authorities will be improved by establishment of contact points on animal transport in each member state. Infringements by transporters and withdrawal of authorisations will be notified to all contact points concerned so as to prevent repeated or serious offenders continuing to operate. Operation and enforcement should be improved as the EU Regulation is directly applicable in all member states. This will improve harmonisation across all member states and avoid inconsistent interpretations that are possible under a Directive.

Further information on the implementation of the rules imposed by Regulation (EC) No. 1/2005 will be available from the DEFRA website: www.defra.gov.uk.

Chapter 22

Law on the Import and Export of Animals

Introduction

Even the complexities of legislation already encountered come nowhere near the convolutions of legal detail associated with the import and export of animals. It would be impossible to do full justice to this area of law in a book such as this. Much of the material is hardly relevant to those who deal with laboratory animals – for example, the niceties of the legality of importing bees from Fiji (*Implementation of the Balai Directive (92/65) in Great Britain*, paragraph 11; an annex from the Animal Health and Veterinary Group, August 1993). Other examples of the minutiae of regulations concerning animals imported into the UK are found in the Animals and Animal Products (Import and Export) Regulations 1993:

> 'Schedule 5
> 3 (a) The official health certification accompanying all cattle imported into Great Britain from Canada must state the animals do not originate from herds in the geographic region of the Okanagan Valley in British Columbia as defined by Commission Decision 88/212/EEC on health protection measures concerning bluetongue in respect of Canada (OJ No. L95, 13/4/88 p. 21). Cattle imported from Canada may only land in Great Britain between 1st February and 15th April inclusive.'

or

> '11 (b) The official health certificate accompanying all swine imported into Great Britain from Bulgaria must state that the animals comply with the requirements of Commission Decision 93/24/EEC on 11/12/1992 concerning additional guarantees relating to Aujesky's disease for pigs destined to member states or regions free of the disease (OJ No. l6 25.1.93 p. 16).'

Such examples serve to make the point that in this chapter we will be merely viewing the very tip of the iceberg, and that indeed from afar. A reader might rightly argue that it is hardly worth doing, but there may be some who are interested in this arcane subject and some laboratory animals do come from or go abroad. In fact the above information could easily now be obsolete. This legislation is extremely fluid depending on the vagaries of politics, the variable interests of commerce and the ever changing pattern of animal health. In the context of the Balai Directive, there are continuous negotiations on animal trade between the EU and so-called third countries (listed countries outside the EU) which affect all member states within the Union such as the Irish Republic and the UK. Special concessions, for example, may be granted to Latvia by Brussels as regards goats or a special concession may be granted as regards mules from Moldavia. Such obscure agreements may have implications for an Irish purchaser of a goat or a horse dealer in Devon.

There is only one practical answer in the presence of such a plethora (the unkind might say quagmire) of regulatory material – availability of an authoritative source or an appropriate address (see Appendix of Useful Addresses).

In Northern Ireland, relevant information should be available from the Northern Ireland Office at Stormont. This may vary a little from mainland legislation. Crown dependencies, such as Jersey or the Isle of Man usually have comparable legislation to that in England and Wales.

The times are changing and devolution marches on. Some of the addresses in the Appendix may be altered. Indeed, an official Notice issued by the Department of the Environment Wildlife Trade Licensing Branch (as revised May 1995) on Import and Export Control passes the buck, stating:

'2. Although care has been taken in the preparation of this Notice, it is intended for guidance only and is not an authoritative interpretation of the law. On points of law, applicants should obtain their own independent legal advice.'

However, even in what rightly could be regarded as the appropriate professional circles the law is not always as crystal clear as we might hope. Expert lawyers can come up with wrong answers. Solicitors have in fact been found guilty of negligence when following counsel's advice. The courts have held that a solicitor ought to have realised that the advice given by counsel was wrong or that the solicitor has chosen the wrong barrister for the job (*Law Notes*, September 1992, col. 1, p. 23, Butterworth, London).

Quarantine

Quarantine may be described as the isolation of individuals suspected of possibly carrying infectious material, for a period that is reckoned to be longer than the supposed period of incubation of the feared disease. Pieces of legislation appearing to tackle the problem directly are such Orders as:

- Rabies Virus Order 1979
- Specified Animal Pathogen Order 1993

The Rabies Virus Order applies to lyssa virus of the family Rhabdoviridae (other than that contained in a medicinal product which may be imported under the

Medicines Act 1968). It is even an offence to keep or use the rabies virus. Both are modern examples of a long line of orders stretching back to the reign of King John (1199–1216) which were intended to protect a farmer's property from destruction by disease.

The salient piece of legislation in the twentieth century was the Rabies (Importation of Dogs, Cats and Other Mammals) Order 1974 with its various amendments in 1984, 1986 and the important 1994 amendment taking into account the Balai Directive. The Balai Directive allows for commercial importation of cats and dogs under stringent conditions of place of origin and certainty of vaccination. The Rabies Act of 1974 was mainly concerned with the control of a possible outbreak of rabies in this country.

The spread of rabies from animals to humans is controlled jointly by DEFRA and the Department of Health. Plans for dealing with this aspect of rabies control are contained in the Memorandum on Rabies issued by the Department of Health.

UK quarantine laws still apply with respect to animals coming from countries outside the European Union. There may be some specific regulations regarding such matters as certification if, as already mentioned, the EU has specific agreements with the third country from which the animals are obtained. If such agreements exist there could also be European stipulations as regards the export of animals or particular species to that country.

UK quarantine regulations still apply to any animals coming from another member state of the EU if the animal does not conform with exemptions allowed for under the Balai Directive (see below), or if the animal is a pet, or if the animal is not being transferred in the course of trade.

The detailed provisions of UK quarantine law come from the Rabies (Importation of Dogs, Cats and Other Mammals) Order 1974 and its amendments. This legislation controls not only the movement of imported animals, but also contacts with imported animals, vaccination of dogs and cats, and action to be taken regarding illegally landed animals or stray animals in ports and airports as listed in Schedule 2 of the Order. There are strict provisions to prevent animals on board boats in British harbours from coming into contact with animals ashore. Offences against the Rabies Order carry heavy penalties including the destruction of the animal. Special arrangements may be made for animals travelling to and from the UK for the purposes of sport, entertainment or breeding.

The term of quarantine for most species is six months. In the case of the vampire bat it is perpetual. Rabies affects bats as well as terrestrial animals. A strain of rabies called European Bat Lyssavirus (EBLV 2) has been found in Daubenton's bats in the UK on four occasions. There was also a fatal human case of rabies in Scotland in December 2002. For most birds the period of quarantine is 37 days. In some cases its duration may be specified in the import licence.

The landing of imported animals into the UK is supervised by HM Revenue & Customs. Quarantine must be spent at DEFRA-approved premises. There must be regular veterinary inspection. Vehicles for the transport of quarantine animals must be DEFRA-approved.

Some orders on importation are still made independently of EU Directives. The Importation of Animals Order 1977 was amended by the Importation of Animals (Amendment) Order 1996. It was short and consisted only of an extension of the definition of 'animals':

> 'In the definition of "animals" in article 2(1) of the Importation of Animals Order 1977(b), for the words "ruminating animals and swine", there shall be substituted the words "ruminating animals, swine and elephants".'

Prominent among the exemptions to the quarantine regulations is the Pet Travel Scheme (PETS). This scheme allows pet dogs, cats and ferrets from certain countries to enter the UK without quarantine as long as they meet the rules. It also means that people in the UK can take their dogs, cats and ferrets to other European Union (EU) countries, and return with them to the UK. They can also, having taken their dogs, cats and ferrets to certain non-EU countries, bring them back to the UK without the need for quarantine.

PETS was introduced, for dogs and cats, for certain European countries on 28/2/2000. EU Regulation on the movement of pet animals extended the scheme to include ferrets, increased the number of qualifying (listed) countries and introduced an EU pet passport and third-country veterinary certificate.

EC Regulation 998/2003 on the non-commercial movement of pet animals applied from 3/7/2004. The Regulation, operated in the UK as the Pet Travel Scheme (PETS) allows cats, dogs, ferrets, domestic rabbits and rodents which comply with certain conditions and are from qualifying countries only to enter the UK without going into quarantine.

The EU Regulation on the movement of pet animals also covers birds (except certain poultry), ornamental tropical fish, invertebrates (except bees and crustaceans), amphibians and reptiles. Persons using PETS must abide by all the rules of the scheme, for example as regards specific countries and specified routes. Details are available from DEFRA at www.defra.gov.uk.

Horse Passports (England) Regulations 2004 require all owners to obtain a passport for each horse they own. This includes ponies, donkeys and other equidae, but excludes zebras and other non-domestic equidae. Owners are not able to sell, buy, export, slaughter for human consumption, or use for the purposes of competition or breeding a horse which does not have a passport. Veterinary authorities have stressed the importance of this measure for horse welfare in the UK. Scotland, Wales and Northern Ireland have similar legislation.

The importing of invertebrates is covered by UK law. A plant health import legislation guide for importers entitled *Importing Invertebrates* was published by MAFF in 1988. The most important sentence in the guide is: 'If in doubt seek help from the Department concerned' – now, of course, DEFRA (website as above).

It is forbidden to import plant and tree pests. The controls apply both to import and export of listed invertebrate pests. It is an offence to knowingly keep, release, sell, exchange or give away any live invertebrate that is a plant or tree pest.

There is always the possibility that even with respect to invertebrates there may be a need to consider law originating outside the UK. The European Commission

Regulations 3626/82 and 3418/83 give the provisions of CITES legal force throughout the European Community and set out the rules for importing species into and exporting species from the Union. For some species, CITES Regulations also impose strict trade controls and restrictions on sale and display. The Endangered Species (Import and Export) Act 1976 has largely been superseded by the EC CITES Regulations. DEFRA will provide details and lists of animals which cannot be imported or are protected by European or international conservation controls. This data is regularly revised.

The Balai [catch-all] Directive

'Balai' (from the French) well merits the translation 'catch-all' for it truly affects all aspects of free trade within and into the European Union. The movement of animals, if involved in commerce, is directly affected by the Regulation stemming from this Directive (92/65/EEC). UK regulations on the import and export of animals have been moulded by this Directive. The comprehensive Animals and Animal Products (Import and Export) Regulations 1993 implemented the Council Directive 90/425/EEC concerning veterinary and zootechnical checks applicable in intra-Community trade in certain live animals and products with a view to completion of the single market; and Council Directive 91/496/EEC laid down principles governing the organisation of veterinary checks on animals entering the Community from third countries. The Animals and Animal Products (Import and Export) Regulations 1995 were written in the light of the Balai Directive (refer to Article 11 of these Regulations). Various other Directives and Decisions of the European Commission have influenced the formation of these Regulations, which have been continually amended. For example, the Animals and Animal Products (Import and Export) (England) (Amended) Regulations 2007 No. 3.

Among all this array of legal technicalities one salient piece of legislation must be stressed and clearly presented. Because of an opt-out obtained by the UK government, part of the quarantine legislation remains intact in Schedule 6 of the Animals and Animal Products (Import and Export) Regulations 1995:

> 'The Rabies (Importation of Dogs, Cats and Other Mammals) Order 1974 shall continue to apply to all carnivores, primates and bats. It shall continue to apply to the importation of all other animals unless such animals are imported by way of trade and can be shown to have been born on the holding of origin and kept in captivity since birth.'

Schedule 6 lists other minor opt-outs from the Balai Directive as regards birds, fish, embryos, ova and semen. It should be consulted by interested parties. It is the clearest official source material in the whole of this legislative maze.

Significant points from the Balai Directive

The scope of the Directive

The Balai Directive lays down specific rules and conditions for:

- apes
- ungulates (including zoo ruminants, deer and suidae)
- birds (other than poultry)
- bees
- rabbits and hares
- ferrets, mink and foxes
- cats and dogs
- other rabies-susceptible species (a true 'catch-all' Directive)
- semen, ova and embryos of the ovine, caprine and equine species and ova and embryos of swine (Articles 5–11).

The Directive lays down the animal health requirements governing intra-community trade in, and imports into the Community of, animals, semen, ova and embryos not subject to animal health requirements laid down elsewhere in specific Community rules.

It does not cover movements of animals or genetic material inside a member state or the movement of pet animals. Any animals such as reptiles, amphibians, and insects (other than bees) not subject to specific rules or animal health rules laid down in other EC Directives, may be traded freely within the Community. In fact, as a general rule, member states are not permitted to prohibit or restrict trade in animals within the Community that is not covered by Community rules (Articles 3–4). However, in the case of imports from third countries, all consignments must be accompanied by approved certification.

A statement in Article 10 confirms Schedule 6 of the Animals and Animal Products (Import and Export) Regulations 1995:

> 'The United Kingdom and Ireland can maintain their quarantine regulations for all carnivores without prejudice to the provisions for cats and dogs, primates, bats and other rabies-susceptible species covered by the Directive which have not been born on the holding of origin and kept in captivity since birth.'

The Directive was published in the *Official Journal of the European Communities*, No. L268, pp. 54–72 (14/9/1992). Copies are obtainable from the Stationery Office.

Special provisions regarding various groups of animals

(i) Apes

Intra-community trade in apes will be generally confined to animals consigned to and from bodies, institutes and centres approved by the competent authorities of member states in accordance with criteria laid down in the Directive. However, by way of derogation member states may authorise acquisition of apes belonging to an individual. All consignments will have to be accompanied by a health certificate corresponding to the model laid down in the Directive (Article 5).

Imports of apes into Great Britain from other member states will be permitted without the animals going into quarantine if they are consigned from and to an approved body, institute or centre.

(ii) Cats and dogs

When cats and dogs which have been born, and have remained, in a single rabies-free premises, have been vaccinated, and where the subsequent blood test has proved that vaccination has been effective, such animals may be exported to the UK without quarantine. They must be identified in accordance with detailed rules and have full veterinary records, and be carried in an approved manner (Article 10).

(iii) Birds

In the case of importation of birds, it would seem that it would be possible to obtain permission to bring them into the UK without quarantine if the birds have been resident in the member state or in quarantine in that member state for a period of at least 35 days and are accompanied by full health certification (Article 7).

(iv) Lagomorphs

Lagomorphs born on the holding of origin and kept in captivity since birth may be imported into Great Britain from another member state, providing that they are accompanied on importation by all the appropriate certification (e.g. that the holding of origin has been free from rabies for at least one month (Article 9)).

(v) Other rabies-susceptible animals (e.g. rats and mice)

If they can be shown to have been born on the holding of origin and kept in captivity since birth, these animals may be imported into Great Britain from another member state providing that they are accompanied on importation by a certificate completed by the exporter confirming that status, that the animals do not show any obvious signs of disease at the time of export, and that the premises of origin are not subject to any animal health restrictions (Article 10).

(vi) Genetic material

Intra-community trade in semen, ova and embryos of the ovine, caprine and equine species and ova and embryos of swine is permitted subject to collection and processing in approved centres or by approved terms, under conditions laid down in the Directive. Consignments must be accompanied by a health certificate (Article 11).

Balai approval

The Directive provides for the approval of bodies, institutes or centres where animals are kept:

- for display and the education of the public, or
- for conservation of the species or scientific research

and which intend either to export to or import from other member states any animal covered by the Directive.

Third countries

Animals, semen, ova and embryos may only be imported from an approved third country whose name appears on a list drawn up by the Community. All such consignments must be accompanied by a health certificate agreed by Standing Veterinary Committee procedure confirming that the animals or genetic material meets any specific animal health requirements laid down by the Community. Outside the scope of this list of third countries, existing national import rules apply (Articles 17–18).

Balai and animal exportation

The main concern of the Directive is the promotion of free trade without let or hindrance, so its controls on export are less severe than its stipulations on importation of animals. This aspect is not of so much concern to us because animals are going out of this country and our quarantine laws are not involved. Here the emphasis of the Directive is on export into member states either from other member states, from third countries with agreement or from any other states. The rules of the Directive stress the importance of the provision of extensive certification which must be bilingual in nature.

Export of animals in UK law

The Animal Health Act 1981 restricts the export of horses and other animals and makes provision for those which are exported.

The Animal Health Act stipulates that proper arrangements for conveying animals to their destination must be made. A route plan should be provided if appropriate. There should be out-of-hours emergency contact numbers of at least two people to avoid animals being left waiting too long before being collected from the point of arrival.

It must be realised when exporting animals that most countries in the world have a substantial network of import restrictions. Very few species of animals, their products or parts can be exported without passing through government controls of the country of destination. These often include an importation licence, comprehensive health certification, maybe quarantine in the country of departure and subsequent quarantine in the country of destination, and customs procedures on arrival.

A(SP)A and importation

The Animal Procedures Committee expressed their concern about importation of animals within the context of A(SP)A. In their 1997 Report (p. 35, vii) they express their intention to:

'Investigate what can be done to ensure that, when animals are acquired from overseas, they are obtained from suitable sources and journey times are minimised.'

The Home Office Inspectorate is therefore involved with the importation of laboratory animals, particularly primates. In the case of Schedule 2 animals, it is obvious that special permission must be obtained from the Secretary of State to acquire such animals because from the very fact that they originate outside the UK, they could not have come from a designated establishment.

Researchers involved with importing animals, besides taking the obvious step of consulting the Inspector on the matter, should take note of the following Order: the revised import conditions for rodents and lagomorphs for research under the Rabies (Importation of Dogs, Cats and other Mammals (England) (Amendment) Order 2004.

This Order allows for rodents or lagomorphs going to research to be imported, and subject to various conditions to be imported without quarantine. An import licence issued by DEFRA is still required and conditions attached to this licence include:

- Animals must have been born and bred in captivity.
- Animals must not have been vaccinated against rabies with a live vaccine in the six months preceding export.
- Animals must be accompanied by a certificate signed by the responsible veterinary or medical supervisor or other appropriately qualified responsible person of the originating establishment stating that:
  (a) Prior to export animals have been in the research/breeding establishment for not less than 15 days.
  (b) The colony has been closed for not less than 15 days or the animals to be exported have been caged and separated or isolated from any new introductions for a period of 15 days.
  (c) For the 12 months prior to shipment, the animals have been kept in an establishment(s) where no case of rabies was reported for at least 12 months.
  (d) No experiments with rabies or rabies-related virus have been carried out in the establishment of origin during the 12 months preceding shipment.
  (e) The animals showed no clinical signs of rabies on the day of shipment.

Other conditions relating to transport of animals, designated ports or airports, accompanying paperwork, etc. apply as in the original legislation.

Note: Forms and conditions associated with the import of rodent embryos, ova and semen are to be obtained from DEFRA: http://www.defra.gov.uk/corporate/reglat/forms/rabies/index.htm

As far as the Home Office is concerned the offspring of imported embryos should be coded in the annual return of procedures according to their place of birth, that is as UK animals.

Standard Conditions

The standard conditions attached to certificates and licences appear in guidance as appendices B, C, D and E.

Appendix A in guidance is the text of the Animals (Scientific Procedures) Act 1986.

Appendix B: Standard conditions: designated scientific procedure establishments

The authority conferred by this certificate is subject to the following conditions. Certificates may be revoked or varied for a breach of conditions.

For the purpose of these conditions, 'Inspector' means a person appointed under the terms of section 18 of the Animals (Scientific Procedures) Act 1986.

1. The areas within the establishment approved by the Secretary of State for the housing of protected animals or the performance of regulated procedures shall be maintained to at least the standards set out in the Home Office Code of Practice for the Housing and Care of Animals used in Scientific Procedures, except where variations are authorised by the Secretary of State.

2. Unless authorised by the Secretary of State, there shall be no variation of the use of the approved areas of the designated establishment that may have adverse consequences for the welfare of the protected animals held.

3. Unless otherwise authorised by the Secretary of State:
   (i) Only the types of protected animals specified in the certificate may be kept in the establishment for use in experimental or other scientific purposes; and
   (ii) these animals may only be kept and used in the areas listed in the schedule to the certificate.

4. The establishment shall be appropriately staffed at all times to ensure the well-being of the protected animals.

5. Unless otherwise authorised in a project licence, regulated procedures shall not be carried out on any of the types of animal listed in Schedule 2 of the Animals (Scientific Procedures) Act 1986 (as amended) unless the animals have been bred at or obtained from an establishment designated by a certificate issued under section 7 of that Act.

   Furthermore, unless otherwise authorised in a project licence, regulated procedures shall not be carried out on cats or dogs unless the animals have been bred at *and* obtained from a breeding establishment designated by a certificate issued under section 7 of the Animals (Scientific Procedures) Act 1986.

6. Records shall be maintained, in a format acceptable to the Secretary of State, of the source, use and final disposal of all protected animals accommodated in the establishment for experimental or other scientific purposes. Such records shall, on request, be submitted to the Secretary of State or made available to an Inspector. The certificate holder shall, on request, submit to the Secretary of State a summary report, in a form specified by the Secretary of State, of the source, use and disposal of all protected animals accommodated in the establishment for experimental or other specific purposes.

7. Records shall be maintained, in a format acceptable to the Secretary of State and under the supervision of the Named Veterinary Surgeon, relating to the health of all protected animals kept for experimental or other scientific purposes and accommodated or used in the establishment. These records shall be readily available, on request, for examination by an Inspector.

8. For the purpose of this condition, 'marked' means clearly identifiable by a method acceptable to the Secretary of State.
    (i)   Each cat, dog and non-human primate in the establishment which is used, or intended for use, in regulated procedures shall be marked, and particulars of the identity and origin of all such animals shall be entered into the records referred to in 6 above.
    (ii) Every cat, dog and non-human primate in the establishment which is used, or intended for use, in regulated procedures shall be marked before it is weaned except where:
          a) the animal is transferred from one establishment to another before it is weaned; and
          b) it is not practicable to mark it beforehand,
          in which case, the receiving establishment shall maintain records attesting the identity and origin of the animal's mother until the animal is marked.
    (iii) Any unmarked cat, dog or non-human primate which is taken into the establishment after weaning shall be marked as soon as possible.

9. In accordance with the Code of Practice for the Housing and Care of Animals used in Scientific Procedures, all protected animals must at all times be provided with adequate care and accommodation appropriate to their type or species. Any restrictions on the extent to which such an animal can satisfy its physiological and ethological needs shall be kept to the absolute minimum; and the health and well-being of protected animals, and the environmental conditions in all parts of the establishment where protected animals are kept, shall be checked at least once daily by competent persons. Arrangements shall be made to ensure that any suffering or defect discovered is remedied as quickly as possible.

9A. The certificate holder shall nominate and be responsible for the performance of named persons, acceptable to the Secretary of State, as required by section 6(5) of the Animals (Scientific Procedures) Act 1986.

10. The person(s) named in the certificate as responsible for the day-to-day care of animals (the Named Animal Care and Welfare Officer(s)) shall ensure that any protected animal which is not the immediate responsibility of any personal licensee and which is found to be in severe pain or severe distress which cannot be alleviated shall be promptly and humanely killed by a competent person using an appropriate method under Schedule 1 to the Act or another method authorised in the certificate of designation.

11. In any case where it appears to the Named Veterinary Surgeon(s) or to the Named Animal Care and Welfare Officer(s) responsible for the day-to-day care of the animals that the health or the welfare of a protected animal kept for experimental or other scientific purposes at the establishment gives rise to concern, he or she shall notify the personal licensee responsible for the animal. If there are no such licensees or if one is not available, the Named Veterinary Surgeon or the Named Animal Care and Welfare Officer responsible for the day-to-day care of the animal shall take steps to ensure that the animal is cared for or, if necessary, humanely killed by a competent person using an appropriate method under Schedule 1 to the Act or another method authorised in the certificate of designation.

12. Arrangements to ensure that animals are given adequate care must be made in the event that the Named Persons referred to in 9A above are not available for any reason.

13. Adequate security measures shall be maintained to prevent the escape of protected animals and to prevent intrusions by unauthorised persons.

14. Quarantine and acclimatisation facilities shall be provided and used as necessary.

15. Adequate precautions against fire shall be maintained at all times.

16. The certificate holder shall take all reasonable steps to prevent the performance of unauthorised procedures in the establishment, and make adequate and effective provision for regular and effective liaison with and between those entrusted with responsibilities under the Act and with others who have responsibility for the welfare of the protected animals kept there.

17. In any case where it is intended to kill a protected animal that has been kept at the establishment for scientific purposes but is not required to be killed under the terms of a project licence, the method of killing employed must be one that is appropriate under Schedule 1 to the Act or otherwise authorised in the certificate. The certificate holder shall ensure that a person competent to kill animals in accordance with this condition is available at all times. A register shall be maintained of those deemed by the certificate holder to be competent to kill by Schedule 1 methods and by any other method specified in the certificate; these methods of killing shall only be entrusted to and performed by such people. The register shall, on request, be submitted to the Secretary of State or made available to an Inspector.

18. Inspectors shall be provided with access at all reasonable times to all parts of the establishments which are concerned with the use, holding or care of protected animals.

19. The certificate holder shall take steps to provide such education and training as is necessary for all licensees and others responsible for the welfare and care of protected animals at the establishment.

20. The certificate holder shall notify the Secretary of State of any proposed change in:
     (i)   the title of the designated establishment; or
     (ii)   the full name of the certificate holder; or
     (iii) the full name(s) and qualifications of the Named Animal Care and Welfare Officer(s) responsible for the day-to-day care of the protected animals; or
     (iv)   the full name(s) and qualifications of the Named Veterinary Surgeon(s); or
     (v)   the areas appearing on the Schedule of Premises for the designated establishment or the class of use within those areas; or
     (vi)   the types of protected animals to be used, or kept for use in regulated procedures.

21. The certificate holder shall notify the Secretary of State of the death of a project licence holder within seven days of its coming to his or her knowledge when, unless the Secretary of State directs otherwise, the project licence shall continue in force for 28 days from the date of notification. The certificate holder will, during that period assume responsibility for ensuring compliance with the terms and conditions of the project licence.

22. A protected animal which, having been subjected to a completed series of regulated procedures, is kept alive shall continue to be kept at the designated establishment under the supervision of a veterinary surgeon or other suitably qualified person unless:
    (i)   it is moved, with the authority of the Secretary of State, to another designated establishment;
    (ii) a veterinary surgeon certifies, and the Secretary of State accepts, that it will not suffer if it ceases to be kept at the designated establishment; or
    (iii) its re-use in another procedure is authorised by the Secretary of State.

23. The certificate holder is required to have instituted, and to maintain, local ethical review processes acceptable to the Secretary of State. Details of the processes and records of the outputs from the processes shall, on request, be submitted to the Secretary of State or made available to an Inspector. Any substantial changes to the processes that are proposed must be submitted to the Secretary of State for approval.

24. A copy of these conditions shall be readily available for consultation by all licensees and named persons in the establishment.

25. The certificate holder shall pay such periodical fees to the Secretary of State as may be prescribed by or determined in accordance with an Order made by him.

26. The certificate remains the property of the Secretary of State, and shall be surrendered to him on request.

Appendix C: Standard conditions: designated breeding and supplying establishments

The authority conferred by this certificate is subject to the following conditions. Certificates may be revoked or varied for a breach of conditions.

For the purpose of these conditions, 'Inspector' means a person appointed under the terms of section 18 of the Animals (Scientific Procedures) Act 1986.

1. In these conditions the word 'animal' means any of the species listed in Schedule 2 to the Act (as amended).

1A. Unless otherwise authorised by the Secretary of State, only those types of animal specified in the certificate, and intended for use in experimental or other scientific procedures, may be bred or kept at the establishment. Furthermore, they may only be bred and kept in the areas listed in the schedule to the certificate.

2. The areas of the establishment approved by the Secretary of State for the housing of protected animals shall be maintained to at least the standards set out in the Home Office Code of Practice for the Housing and Care of Animals in Designated Breeding and Supplying Establishments, except where variations are authorised by the Secretary of State.

3. Unless authorised by the Secretary of State, there shall be no variation of the use of the approved areas of the designated establishment which may have adverse consequences for the welfare of the protected animals held.

4. The establishment shall be appropriately staffed at all times to ensure the well-being of the animals.

5. Records shall be maintained, in a format acceptable to the Secretary of State, of the source, use and final disposal of all protected animals bred, kept for breeding or kept for subsequent supply for use for experimental or other scientific purposes. These shall, on request, be submitted to the Secretary of State or made available to an Inspector. The certificate holder shall, on request, submit to the Secretary of State a summary report, in a form specified by the Secretary of State, of the source, use and disposal of all protected animals bred, kept for breeding or kept for subsequent supply for use for experimental or other scientific purposes.

6. A health record relating to all protected animals bred, kept for breeding or kept for subsequent supply for use for experimental or other scientific purposes and accommodated in the establishment shall be maintained in a format acceptable to the Secretary of State and under the supervision of the Named Veterinary Surgeon. This record shall, on request, be submitted to the Secretary of State or made available to an Inspector.

7. For the purpose of this condition, 'marked' means clearly identifiable by a method acceptable to the Secretary of State.
   (i)   Each cat, dog and non-human primate in the establishment which is intended for use in regulated procedures shall be marked, and particulars of the identity and origin of all such animals shall be entered into the records referred to in 5 above.
   (ii) Every cat, dog and non-human primate kept in the establishment which is intended for use in regulated procedures shall be marked before it is weaned except where:
         a)   the animal is transferred from one establishment to another before it is weaned; and
         b)   it is not practicable to mark it beforehand,
         in which case, the receiving establishment shall maintain records attesting the identity and origin of the animal's mother until the animal is marked.
   (iii) Any unmarked cat, dog or non-human primate which is taken into the establishment after weaning shall be marked as soon as possible.

8. Unless otherwise authorised by the Secretary of State, animals must be obtained from establishments designated under section 7 of the Animals (Scientific Procedures) Act 1986.

9. In accordance with the Code of Practice for the Housing and Care of Animals in Designated Breeding and Supplying Establishments, all protected animals must at all times be provided with adequate care and accommodation appropriate to their type or species. Any restrictions on the extent to which such an animal can satisfy its physiological and ethological needs shall be kept to a minimum; and the health and well-being of protected animals and the environmental conditions in all parts of the establishment where protected animals are kept shall be checked at least once daily by competent persons and arrangements made to ensure that any suffering or defect discovered is remedied as quickly as possible.

9A. The certificate holder shall nominate and be responsible for the performance of named persons, acceptable to the Secretary of State, as required by section 7(5) of the Animals (Scientific Procedures) Act 1986.

10. The person named in the certificate as responsible for the day-to-day care of animals (the Named Animal Care and Welfare Officer) shall ensure that any animal which is found to be in severe pain or severe distress which cannot be alleviated shall be promptly and humanely killed by a competent person using an appropriate method under Schedule 1 to the Act or another method authorised in the certificate of designation.

11. In any case where it appears to the Named Veterinary Surgeon or to the Named Animal Care and Welfare Officer responsible for the day-to-day care of the animals that the health or the welfare of an animal at the establishment gives rise to concern, he or she shall take steps to ensure that the animal is either cared for or, if necessary, humanely killed by a competent person using an appropriate method under Schedule 1 to the Act or another method authorised in the certificate of designation.

12. Arrangements to ensure that animals are given adequate care must be made in the event that the named persons referred to in condition 9A above are not available for any reason.

13. Adequate security measures shall be maintained to prevent the escape of protected animals and to prevent intrusions by unauthorised persons.

14. Quarantine and acclimatisation facilities shall be provided and used as necessary.

15. Adequate precautions against fire shall be maintained at all times.

16. In any case where it is intended to kill a protected animal which has been bred, kept for breeding or kept for subsequent supply for use for experimental or other scientific purposes the method of killing employed must be one which is appropriate under Schedule 1 to the Act or otherwise authorised in the certificate. The certificate holder shall ensure that a person competent to kill animals in accordance with this condition is available at all times. A register shall be maintained of those deemed by the certificate holder to be competent to kill by Schedule 1 methods and by any other method specified in the certificate; these methods of killing shall only be entrusted to and performed by such people. The register shall, on request, be submitted to the Secretary of State or made available to an Inspector.

17. Inspectors shall be provided with access at all reasonable times to all parts of the establishment relating to the holding or care of protected animals.

18. The certificate holder shall notify the Secretary of State of any proposed change in:
     (i)   the title of the designated establishment; or
     (ii)   the full name of the certificate holder; or
     (iii) the full name(s) and qualifications of the Named Animal Care and Welfare Officer(s) responsible for the day-to-day care of the protected animals; or
     (iv)   the full name(s) and qualifications of the Named Veterinary Surgeon(s); or
     (v)   the areas appearing on the Schedule of Premises for the designated establishment; or
     (vi)   the types of protected animal to be bred or kept for use on regulated procedures.

19. The certificate holder shall take steps to provide such education and training as is necessary to those entrusted with the care and welfare of protected animals at the establishment and to ensure that adequate and effective provision is made for regular and effective communication with and between those entrusted with responsibilities under the Act and with others who have responsibility for the welfare of the animals kept there.

20. The certificate holder is required to have instituted, and to maintain, local ethical review processes acceptable to the Secretary of State. Details of the processes and records of the outputs from the processes shall, on request, be submitted to the Secretary of State or made available to an Inspector. Any substantial changes to the processes must be submitted to the Secretary of State for approval.

21. A copy of these conditions shall be readily available for consultation by all persons in the establishment responsible for the health, care and welfare of animals.

22. The certificate holder shall pay such periodical fees to the Secretary of State as may be prescribed by or determined in accordance with an Order made by him.

23. The certificate remains the property of the Secretary of State and shall be surrendered to him on request.

Appendix D: Standard conditions: project licences

The authority conferred by this licence is subject to the following conditions. Licences may be revoked or varied for a breach of conditions.

In addition, breaches of conditions 1 to 5 may be criminal offences under the Act.

For the purpose of these conditions, 'Inspector' means a person appointed under the terms of section 18 of the Animals (Scientific Procedures) Act 1986.

1. The project licence holder shall not, in pursuit of this programme of work, procure or knowingly permit any person under his or her control to carry out regulated procedures otherwise than in accordance with:
   (i)   the programme of work specified in this licence; and
   (ii) that person's personal licence.

2. Procedures under the authority of the project licence shall be carried out only at the place or places specified in the licence, unless their performance elsewhere is authorised by the Secretary of State.

3. No person working under the authority of the project licence shall use any neuro-muscular blocking agent in place of an anaesthetic.

4. No person working under the authority of the project licence shall use any neuro-muscular blocking agent without express authority from the Secretary of State, which must be contained in both the project and personal licences.

5. No animal which has completed a series of regulated procedures for a particular purpose may be used again on the same procedure/protocol, or on another procedure/protocol whether on the same licence or another, without express authority in this project licence.

6. For any procedure, the degree of severity imposed shall be the minimum consistent with the attainment of the objectives of the procedure, and this shall not exceed the

severity limit attached to the procedure. The minimum number of animals of the lowest neurophysiological sensitivity shall be used in procedures causing the least pain, suffering, distress or lasting harm.

6A.   All authorised procedures shall be carried out under general, regional or local anaesthesia unless:
  (i)   anaesthesia would be incompatible with the purposes of the procedures; or
  (ii)   anaesthesia would be more traumatic to the animal concerned than the procedures themselves.

6B.   Except where incompatible with the purposes of the procedures, when an anaesthetised animal suffers considerable pain once the anaesthesia has worn off that animal shall be given pain-relieving treatment in good time or if this is not possible, it shall be promptly killed by a competent person using an appropriate method under Schedule 1 to the Act or another method authorised in the certificate of designation.

6C.   Where, in accordance with 6A above, anaesthesia is not used, analgesics or other appropriate methods must be used appropriately in order to ensure, as far as possible, that pain, suffering, distress and harm are minimised and that, in any event, the animal is not subject to severe pain, distress or suffering.

7.   Except with the authorisation of the Secretary of State:
  (a)   regulated procedures shall not be carried out on any of the animals listed in Schedule 2 to the Animals (Scientific Procedures) Act 1986 (as amended) unless they have been bred at *or* obtained from a breeding or supplying establishment designated by a certificate issued under section 7 of that Act;
  (b)   furthermore, regulated procedures shall not be carried out on cats and dogs unless they have been bred at *and* obtained from a breeding establishment designated by a certificate issued under section 7 of the Animals (Scientific Procedures) Act 1986; and
  (c)   regulated procedures shall not be carried out on protected animals taken from the wild.

7A.   Animals may only be set free into the wild during the course of a procedure with the authority of the Secretary of State. Animals shall not be set free into the wild as part of programmes of work for education and training.

8.   It is the responsibility of the project licence holder to ensure adherence to the severity limits as shown in the listing of procedures/protocols (section 19a) and observance of any other controls described in the procedure/protocol sheets (section 19b). If these constraints appear to have been, or are likely to be breached, the project licence holder shall ensure that the Secretary of State is notified as soon as possible.

9.   It is the responsibility of the project licence holder to maintain a contemporaneous record of all animals on which procedures have been carried out under the authority of the project licence. This record shall show the procedures used and the names of personal licensees who have carried out the procedures. The record shall, on request, be submitted to the Secretary of State or made available to an Inspector.

10.   The project licence holder shall send to the Secretary of State, before 31 January each year (and within 28 days of the licence having expired or been revoked), a report in a form specified by the Secretary of State, giving details of the number of procedures and animals used, and the nature and purpose of the procedures performed under the authority of the project licence during the calendar year.

11. The project licence holder shall maintain a list of publications resulting from the licensed programme of work and a copy of any such publication shall be made available to the Secretary of State on request. The list shall, on request, be submitted to Secretary of State or made available to an Inspector, and it shall be submitted to Secretary of State when the licence is returned to him on expiry or for revocation.

12. The project licence holder shall submit such other reports as the Secretary of State may from time to time require.

13. The project licence holder shall ensure that details of the plan of work and procedures described in sections 18 and 19 of the schedule of this licence, and any additional conditions imposed on those procedures, are known to:
    (i)   all personal licensees performing those procedures;
    (ii) the Named Animal Care and Welfare Officers responsible for the day-to-day care of the animals; and
    (iii) the Named Veterinary Surgeon, on request.

14. The project licence holder shall ensure that the appropriate level of supervision is provided for all personal licensees carrying out regulated procedures under the authority of this licence.

15. The project licence holder must obtain the permission of the Secretary of State before:
    (i)   any animal undergoing regulated procedures is moved from one designated establishment to another; or
    (ii) any animal is released for slaughter; or
    (iii) any animal is released from the controls of the Act,
    unless this is already explicitly authorised by the project licence.

16. At the conclusion of a series of regulated procedures for a particular purpose, protected animals which are suffering, or are likely to suffer, as a result of those procedures shall be promptly and humanely killed:
    (i)   by a competent person using an appropriate method under Schedule 1 to the Act or another method authorised in the certificate of designation; or
    (ii) by another method authorised by the personal licence of the person by whom the animal is killed.

17. If a veterinary surgeon, or other suitably qualified person acceptable to the Secretary of State, determines that animals are not suffering, and are not likely to suffer as a result of the regulated procedures, those animals may be kept at the designated establishment under the supervision of that person.

18. The licence remains the property of the Secretary of State, and shall be surrendered to him on request.

Appendix E: Standard conditions: personal licences

The authority conferred by this licence is subject to the following conditions. Licences may be revoked or varied for a breach of conditions.

In addition, breaches of conditions 1–9 and failure to comply with a requirement under condition 10 may be criminal offences under the Act.

For the purpose of these conditions, 'Inspector' means a person appointed under the terms of section 18 of the Animals (Scientific Procedures) Act 1986.

1. No personal licensee shall carry out a regulated procedure for which authority has not been granted in his or her personal licence.

2. No personal licensee shall use in any regulated procedure any type of protected animal not authorised by his or her personal licence.

3. No personal licensee shall carry out any regulated procedure unless authorised by a project licence.

4. No personal licensee shall carry out any regulated procedure as an exhibition to the general public or carry out any such procedure which is shown live on television for general reception.

5. No personal licensee carrying out any regulated procedure shall use any neuromuscular blocking agent in place of an anaesthetic.

6. No personal licensee shall use any neuromuscular blocking agent without express authority from the Secretary of State which must be contained in both the project and personal licences.

7. Unless otherwise authorised by the Secretary of State in both project and personal licences, personal licensees shall perform the procedures for which they have authority only at the place or places specified in their personal licenses, and only in suitable areas specified in the relevant certificate of designation.

8. The personal licence holder shall arrange for any animal which, at the conclusion of a series of procedures for a particular purpose, is suffering or is likely to suffer adverse effects to be promptly and humanely killed:
    (i)   by a competent person using an appropriate method under Schedule 1 to the Act or another method authorised in the certificate of designation; or
    (ii) by another method authorised by the personal licence of the person by whom the animal is killed.

9. No animal which has completed a series of regulated procedures for a particular purpose may be re-used without express authority in the project licence.

10. If an Inspector requires that an animal must be killed because that Inspector believes that it is undergoing excessive suffering, it must be promptly and humanely killed in accordance with 8(i) or 8(ii) above.

11. It is the responsibility of the personal licensee to ensure that all cages, pens or other enclosures are clearly labelled. The labelling must be such as to enable Inspectors, Named Veterinary Surgeons and Named Animal Care and Welfare Officers to identify the project in which the animals are being used, the regulated procedures which have been performed, and the responsible personal licensee.

12. The personal licensee is entrusted with primary responsibility for the welfare of the animals on which he or she has performed regulated procedures; the personal licensee must ensure that animals are properly monitored and cared for, and must take effective precautions, including the appropriate use of sedatives, tranquillisers, analgesics or anaesthetics, to prevent or reduce to the minimum level consistent with the aims of the procedure any pain, suffering, distress or discomfort caused to the animals used.

13. It is the responsibility of the personal licensee to notify the project licence holder as soon as possible when it appears either that the severity limit of any procedure listed in the project licence (section 19a) or that the constraints upon adverse effects

described in the protocol sheets (section 19b) have been or are likely to be significantly exceeded.

14. In all circumstances where an animal which is being, or has been, subjected to a regulated procedure is in severe pain or severe distress which cannot be alleviated, the personal licensee must ensure that the animal is promptly and humanely killed in accordance with 8(i) or 8(ii) above.

15. It is the responsibility of the personal licensee to ensure that suitable arrangements exist for the care and welfare of animals during any period when the personal licensee is not in attendance.

16. It is the responsibility of the personal licensee to ensure that, whenever necessary, veterinary advice and treatment are obtained for the animals in his or her care.

17. The personal licensee is subjected to such supervision requirements as may be stated on the licence or which the project licence holder may deem necessary in order to ensure that regulated procedures are performed competently.

18. Before any animal, or groups of animals, that has been subjected to procedures is released into the wild, to a farm, or for use as a pet, the personal licensee must ensure that appropriate authority exists in the project licence for the animal or animals to be released.

19. When anaesthesia (whether general, regional or local) is used, it shall be of sufficient depth to prevent the animal from being aware of pain arising during the procedure.

19A. All authorised procedures shall, in accordance with the relevant project licence authorities, be carried out under general, regional or local anaesthesia unless:
(i) anaesthesia would be incompatible with the purpose of the procedures; or
(ii) anaesthesia would be more traumatic to the animal concerned than the procedures themselves.

19B. Except where incompatible with the purposes of the procedures, when an anaesthetised animal suffers considerable pain once the anaesthesia has worn off, the personal licensee shall ensure that, wherever possible, the animal is given pain-relieving treatment in good time or that the animal is promptly and humanely killed in accordance with 8(i) or 8(ii) above.

19C. Where, in accordance with 19A above, anaesthesia is not used, analgesics or other appropriate methods must be used in order to ensure as far as possible that pain, suffering, distress and harm are limited and that in any event the animal is not subject to severe pain, distress or suffering.

20. Personal licensees must take all reasonable steps to ensure appropriate personal and project licence authorities exist before performing regulated procedures, and must be aware of the nature of the current authorities, and the conditions of issue attached to the licences.

21. The personal licensee shall maintain a record of all animals on which procedures have been carried out, including details of supervision and declarations of competence by the project licence holder as appropriate. This record shall be retained for at least five years and shall, on request, be submitted to the Secretary of State or made available to an Inspector.

22. The licence remains the property of the Secretary of State, and shall be surrendered to him on request.

Useful Addresses

Animal Health
DEFRA Area 506
1a Page Street
London SW1P 4PQ

APC (Animal Procedures Committee)
1st Floor
Seacole SW Quarter
2 Marsham Street
London SW1P
Tel: 020 7035 4775
Email: apc.secretariat@homeoffice.gsi.gov.uk
Web: www.apc.gov.uk

Association of the British Pharmaceutical
   Industry (ABPI)
12 Whitehall
London SW1A 2DY
Tel: 020 7930 3477
Web: www.abpi.org.uk

Bioscientific Events Ltd
164 Chislehurst Road
Orpington
Kent BR6 0DT
Tel: 01689 872 953
Email: info@bioscientific.co.uk
Web: www.bioscientific.co.uk

(Conservation)
Joint Nature Conservation Committee
Monkstone House
City Road
Peterborough PE1 1JY
United Kingdom
Email: comment@jncc.gov.uk

Council of Europe
Boitepostale 431R6
F67006 Strasbourg Cedex
France
Tel: 8841 20000
Web: www.consilium.europa.eu

DEFRA (Department for Environment,
   Food & Rural Affairs)
1a Page Street
London SW1 1PQ
Tel: 020 7904 6000
Email: helpline@defra.gsi.gov.uk
Web: defra.gov.uk

DEFRA (Department for
   Environment, Planning &
   Countryside)
Agricultural Dept.
Crown Buildings
Cathays Park
Cardiff CF1 3NQ
Tel: 029 2082 5111
Email: agriculture@wales.gsi.gov.uk
Web: www.wales.gsi.gov.uk

DEFRA NI (Department for Rural Affairs
   Northern Ireland)
Dundonald House
Upper Newtownards Rd
Belfast BT4 3SB
Northern Ireland
Tel: 028 9052 4999
Email: library@dardni.gov.uk
Web: www.dardni.gov.uk

DEFRA Scotland
Scottish Executive Environment & Rural
   Affairs Dept (SEERAD)
Pentland House
47 Robbs Loan
Edinburgh EH14 1TW
Tel: 0131 244 6015
Email: animal.health@scotland.gsi.gov.uk
Web: www.scotland.gov.uk

European Commission Information Office
8 Storey's Gate
London SW1P 3AT
Tel: 020 7973 1992
Web: http://publications.eu.int

European Office for Official Publications
of the European Union
2 rue Mercier
L-2985 Luxembourg
Tel: 352 29 291
Web: http://publications.eu.int

Home Office
Direct Communications Unit
2 Marsham Street
London SW1P 4DF
Tel: 0870 000 1585
Email: public.enquiries@homeoffice.gsi.
gov.uk
Web: scienceandresearch.homeoffice.
gov.uk

IAT (Institute of Animal Technology)
5 South Parade
Summerton
Oxford OX2 7JL
Web: www.iat.org.uk

IATA
GB Nixdorf House
125–135 Staines Road
Hounslow
Middlesex TW3 3JF
Tel: 020 8607 6332

LASA (Laboratory Animals Science
Association)
P O Box 3993
Tamworth B78 3QU
Tel: 01827 259130
Web: www.lasa.co.uk

MHRA Publications Information
Centre
MHRA
Market Towers
1 Nine Elms Lane
London SW8 5NQ
Tel: 020 7084 2000
Email: info@mhra.gsi

MRC (Medical Research Council)
20 Park Crescent
London W1B 1AL
Tel: 020 7636 5422
Email: corporate@headoffice.mrc.ac.uk

NC3Rs
National Centre for the Replacement,
Refinement & Reduction of Animals
in Research
Tel: 020 7670 5331
Email: enquiries@nc3Rs.org.uk

NICE (National Institute for Health &
Clinical Excellence)
71 High Holborn
London WC1V 6NA
Tel: 020 7067 5800
Email: nice@nice.org.uk
Web: www.nice.org.uk

Information may also be available from
Northern Ireland Office
Castle Buildings
Stormont
Belfast BT4 3SG
Tel: 028 9052 0700

Nuffield Council on Bioethics
28 Bedford Square
London
WC1B 3JS
Tel: 020 7681 9619
Web: www.nuffieldbioethics.org

OECD (Organisation for Economic
Cooperation and Development)
2 rue Andre Pascal
75775 Paris Cedex 16
France
Email: webmaster@oecd.org

Office for Official Publications of the
European Union
2 rue Mercier
L-2985 Luxembourg
Tel: 352 29 291

RDS (Research Defence Society)
25 Shaftesbury Avenue
London W1D 7EG
Tel: 020 7287 2818
Email: info@rds-net.org.uk
Web: rds-online.org.uk

UFAW (Universities Federation For
  Animal Welfare)
The Old School
Brewhouse Hill
Wheathampstead
Hertfordshire AL4 8AN
Tel: +44(0) 1582 831 818
Email: ufaw@ufaw.org.uk
Web: www.ufaw.org.uk

Wildlife: Global Wildlife Division
DEFRA
1/17 Temple Quay
Bristol BS1 6EB
Tel: 0117 372 6153
Email: natura.2000@defra.gsi.gov.uk

Libraries and Sources of Information

British Library of Political and Economic
  Science
10 Portugal Street
London WC2A 2HD
Tel: 020 7955 7273

Communitas Europaeae Lex (CELEX)
  available on CD-ROM
Hosts Eurobases
Contex/Limited/Justis: Profile Information

European Commission's Library
  Automated System (ECLAS)
Hosts Eurobases
Commission of the EU
Rue de la Loi 200
B-1049 Brussels

Health and Safety Commission
Rose Court
2 Southwark Bridge
London SE1 9HS
Tel: 020 7717 6000

Jean Monnet House
8 Storey's Gate
London SW1P 3AT
Tel: 020 7973 1900

The British Library
96 Euston Road
St. Pancras
London
NW1 2DB
Tel: +44(0) 20 7412 7332

Useful Websites/Email

Animal Procedures Committee (APC)
www.apc.gov.uk

Animal Scientific Procedures Act (ASPA)
www.homeoffice.gov.uk/comrace/animals/licensing.html

Best Practice
www.lasa.co.uk/bursaries/goodpractice.asp

Bioscientific
www.bioscientific.co.uk

Conservation: Joint Nature Conservation Committee
www.jncc.gov.uk

Conventions (International)
www.unece.org

Cost/Benefit
www.apc.gov.uk/reference/costbenefit.pdf

DEFRA
www.defra.gov.uk

European Convention ETS 123
(Revision of Welfare of Laboratory Animals)
http://.conventions.coe.int/default.asp

European Legislation
CELEX (Communitatis Europaeae Lex) available on CD-ROM
   This covers a compendium of European legislation
   Hosts: Eurobases; Contex Limited/Justis: Profile Information
ECLAS (European Commission's Library Automated System)
   Hosts: Eurobases. Commission of the EU, Rue de Loi 200, B-1049, Brussels.
http://europa.eu.int/eur-lex/lex/Lex Uri Serv/site/en/oj/2005/1003/
100320050105en00010044.pdf

Genetic Manipulation
www.hse.gov.uk/biosafety/gmo/law.htm
http://genome.wellcome.ac.uk/-WTD021014.html

FELASA
Federation of European Laboratory Animal Science Associations
www.felasa.org

Freedom of Information Act (FOI)
www.hmso.gov.uk/acts/2000/20000036.htm

(FOI) Scotland
www.opsi.gov.uk/legislation/scotland/acts2002/20020013.htm

Good Laboratory Practice (GLP)
glp@mhra.gsi.gov.uk

Guidance Notes
www.homeoffice.gov.uk/comrace/animals/legislation.html#legislation

Laboratory Animals (Publications)
www.lal.org.uk

Laboratory Animal Science Association (LASA)
www.lasa.co.uk

Legislation
www.parliament.uk
www.opsi.uk/legislation

Medical Research Council (MRC)
www.mrc.ac.uk

The Medicines and Healthcare Products Regulatory Agency (MHRA)
glp@mhra.gsi.gov.uk

Organisation for Economic Cooperation and Development (OECD)
www.oecd.org/about

Project Licence Forms, Amendments and Abstracts
www.homeoffice.gov.uk/comrace/animals/licensing.html

Pressure Group – Victims of Animal Rights Extremism (VARE)
www.vare.org.uk

Pressure Groups – British Union for the Abolition of Vivisection (BUAV)
www.buav.org

Pressure Groups – Research Defence Society (RDS)
www.rds-online.org.uk

RSPCA
www.rspca.org.uk

3Rs
www.nc3rs.org.uk

Statutory Instruments
www.opsi.gov.uk/stat.htm

Transport
http://europa.eu.int/eur-lex/lex/Lex UriServ/
site/en/oj/2005/1003/100320050105en00010044.pdf

(AATA)
www.aata–animaltransport.org

UFAW
Universities Federation of Animal Welfare
www.ufaw.org.uk

Welfare – Animal Welfare Act
www.defra.gov.uk

NB: Addresses accurate at the time of going to press

Bibliography

Animal Procedures Committee *Annual Reports* 1989 to 2005. HMSO, London.

Animal Procedures Committee Cambridge/BUAV (2006) *Report of Working Group 2005.* APC, London.

Animal Procedures Committee (2006) *Acceptance of Overseas Centres Supplying Non-Human Primates to UK Laboratories.* APC, London.

Animal Procedures Committee (2005) *Report of Statistics Working Group.* HMSO, London.

Animal Procedures Committee (2002) *Report on Biotechnology.* HMSO, London.

Animal Procedures Committee (2001) *Report on Openness.* APC, London.

Animal Procedures Committee (2002) *Report on the Use of Primates under the Animals (Scientific Procedures) Act (1986) – Analysis of Current Trends with Particular Reference to Regulatory Toxicology.* APC, London.

Animal Procedures Committee (2003) *Review of Cost-Benefit Assessment in the Use of Animals in Research.* APC, London.

Animal Welfare – Human Rights: Protecting People from Animal Rights Extremists (2004). Home Office and Department of Trade and Industry, London.

A(SP)A Inspectorate (2004) *Annual Report.* Home Office, London.

Association of Veterinary Teachers and Research Workers (1989) *Guidelines for the Recognition and Assessment of Pain in Animals.* UFAW, Potters Bar.

Barclay, R.J., Herbert, W.J. & Poole, T.B. (1988) *The Disturbance Index: A Behavioural Method of Assessing the Severity of Common Laboratory Procedures on Rodents.* UFAW, Potters Bar.

Burnett, S.W. (2007) *Manual of Animal Technology.* Blackwell Publishing, Oxford.

Biotechnology and Biological Sciences Research Council (1999) *The Use of Animals in Research,* BBSRC Swindon.

Brambell, F.W.R. (1965) *Report of the Advisory Committee on the Welfare of Farm Animals.* HMSO, London.

Broom, D.M. & Johnson, F.G. (1993) Stress and Animal Welfare. Chapman and Hall, London.

Brooman, S. & Legge, D. (1997) *Law Relating to Animals.* Cavendish Publishing, London.

Charter on Licensing and Inspection, replacing the Code of Practice for Licensing and Inspection under the Animals (Scientific Procedures) Act (2000). HMSO, London.

Code of Practice for the Housing and Care of Animals in Designated Breeding and Supplying Establishments (1995). HMSO, London.

Code of Practice for the Housing and Care of Animals used in Scientific Procedures (1989). HMSO, London.

Code of Practice for the Housing and Care of Pigs Intended for use as Xenotransplant Source Animals (1999). HMSO, London.

Code of Practice for the Humane Killing of Animals under Schedule 1 to the Animal (Scientific Procedures) Act 1986 (1996). HMSO, London.

Cooper, M. (1987) *An Introduction to Animal Law.* Academic Press, London.

Council of Europe (1986) *European Convention for the Protection of Vertebrate Animals used for Experimental and other Scientific Purposes.* Strasbourg: Council of Europe. (Obtainable: HMSO).

Council of Europe Working Party (2004) *Draft Guidelines for Accommodation and Care of Animals (ETS N° 123).* Council of Europe, Strasbourg.

de Smith, S.A. (1978) *Constitutional and Administrative Law.* Penguin Books, Harmondsworth.

Department of Health (1989) *Good Laboratory Practice: The UK Compliance Programme.* Department of Health, London.

Dolan, K. (1999) *Ethics, Animals and Science.* Blackwell Science, Oxford.

Dolan, K. & Tobin, S. (1994) *The Animals (Scientific Procedures) Act, Resource Book for Personal Licence Holders.* Spot on Training, London.

European Community (1986) Council Directive 86/609/EEC on the approximation of laws, regulations and administrative provisions of Member States regarding the protection of animals used for experimental and other scientific purposes. OJL.358.

European Federation of Pharmaceutical Industries Associations and European Centre for the Validation of Alternative Methods (2001) *Good Practice Guide to the Administration of Substances and Removal of Blood. Journal of Applied Toxicology* 21: 15–23.

Expert Group on Efficient Regulation (2001) *The Regulation of the Use of Animals in Scientific Procedures.* EGER, PO Box 108, Wilmslow, Cheshire SK9 6FW.

FELASA (1999) *Working party report of the Federation of Laboratory Animal Science Associations working group on education of specialists. Laboratory Animals* 3: 1–15.

FRAME and UFAW (1998) *Selection and Use of Replacement Methods in Animal Experimentation.* UFAW, Potters Bar.

Fraser, A.F. & Broom, D.M. (1990) *Farm Animal Behaviour and Welfare.* Baillière Tindall, London.

GLP Pocket Book (1999) MHRA Publications, 1 Nine Elms Lane, London SW8 5NQ.

Gordon, S., Wallace, J., Cool, A. *et al.* (1997) Reduction of exposure to laboratory animal allergens in the workplace. *Clinical Experimental Allergy* 27: 744–51.

Health and Safety Executive (1990) *What you should know about Allergy to Laboratory Animals.* HSE Books, London.

Health and Safety Executive (2002) *Control of Laboratory Animal Allergy* EH76. HSE Books, Suffolk, http://www.hsebooks.co.uk

Hendriksen, C.F.M. and Morton, D. (1998) *Humane Endpoints in Animal Experiments for Biomedical Research.* The Royal Society of Medicine Press, London.

Hills, A. (2005) *Do Animals Have Rights?* Icon Books, Cambridge.

Hollands, Clive (1980) *Compassion is the Bugler. The Struggle for Animal Rights.* MacDonald, Edinburgh.

Home Office (1987) *Guidelines on Eye Irritation/Corrosion Tests ('Draize' Eye Test) 1987.* Home Office, London.

Home Office (1987) *Supplementary Guidance on Microsurgery Training.* Home Office, London.

Home Office (1990) *Guidelines on A(SP)A and Veterinary Practice.* Home Office, London.

Home Office (1998) *Survey of Welfare Standards for Dogs within Designated Establishments.* The Stationery Office, London.

Home Office (2000) *A Supplementary Note by the Chief Inspector on the Ethical Review Process.* Home Office, London.

Home Office (2000) *Guidance on the Operation of A(SP)A 1986.* HMSO London.

Home Office (2001) *Guidance Note: The Conduct of Regulatory Toxicology and Safety Evaluation Studies.* Home Office, London.

Home Office (2001) *Inspectorate Review of the ERP.* Home Office, London.

Home Office (2001) *Supplementary Guidance: Production of Antibodies as a Service.* Home Office, London.

Home Office (2002) *Guidance Note: Non-Rodent Selection in Pharmaceutical Toxicology.* Home Office, London.

Home Office (2002) *Supplementary Guidance on Education and Training PPL Applications.* Home Office, London.

Home Office (2003) *Guidance Notes on Water and Food Restriction.* Home Office, London.

Home Office Guidance Note (1993) *Projects for Educational Purposes.* Home Office, London.

Home Office Guidance Notes on GM Animals, Home Office, London.

Home Office Statistics of Scientific Procedures on Living Animals, published annually, HMSO, London.

House of Lords (2002) *Select Committee on Animals in Scientific Procedures Report.* HMSO, London.

International Air Transport Association (IATA) *Live Animal Regulations 1998*, 25th edn. IATA, Montreal and Geneva.

International Network for Humane Education (InterNICHE) (2003) 'From Guinea Pig to Computer Mouse' http://www.interniche.org/book.html

Kean, Hilda (1998) *Animal Rights, Political and Social Change in Britain since 1880.* Reaktion Books, London.

Kennedy Committee Report (1997) *Report of the Advisory Group on the Ethics of Xenotransplantation.* The Stationery Office, London.

Laboratory Animal Breeders Association (1993) *Guidelines on the Care and Housing of Animals Bred for Scientific Purposes*, LABA (n.p.)

LaFollette, H. & Shanks, N. (1996) *Dilemmas of Animal Experimentation.* Routledge, London.

Langley, G. (1989) *Animal Experimentation: The Consensus Changes.* Macmillan Press, Basingstoke.

LASA (1998) *The Ethical Review Process in Academia.* LASA, Tamworth.

LASA (2005) 'Guidance on the Transport of Laboratory Animals'. *Laboratory Animals* 39: 1–39.

LASA Working Party (1990) 'The assessment and control of the severity of scientific procedures on laboratory animals'. *Laboratory Animals* 24: 97–130.

LAVA (1998) *The Veterinary Surgeons Act 1966 and the Animals (Scientific Procedures) Act 1986 – a conflict of legislative requirements.* LAVA Position Paper, LAVA, London.

LAVA (2001) *Guidance on the Discharge of Animals from the A(SP)A.* Obtainable from Agenda Resource Management, PO Box 24, Hull HU1 28Y.

Lembeck, F. (1989) *Scientific Alternatives to Animal Experiments.* Ellis Horwood, Chichester.

Linzey, W. (1984) *Animal Rights.* SCM Press, London.

Littlewood Committee (1965) *Report of the Departmental Committee on Experiments on Animals.* HMSO, London.

Live Animal Regulation, 19th edn. International Air Transport Association, Montreal and Geneva. Published annually.

Lund, V. (1997) 'Postgraduate teaching in farm animal welfare and ethics'. *Animal Welfare* 6: 105–21.

Lynam, Shevawn (1975) *Humanity Dick. A Biography of Richard Martin M.P. 1754–1834.* Hamish Hamilton, London.

MacDonald, Melody (1994) *Caught in the Act: The Feldberg Investigation.* Jon Carpenter, Oxford.

Marsh, N. & Haywood, S. (1985) *Animal Experimentation.* FRAME, London.

McMillan, F.D. (ed) (2004) *Mental Health and Well-being in Animals.* Blackwell, Oxford.

Morton, D. & Griffiths, P. (1985) 'Guidelines on the recognition of pain, distress and discomfort in experimental animals and a hypothesis for assessment'. *Veterinary Record*, 20 April.

Moss, Arthur M. (1961) *Valiant Crusader. The History of the RSPCA. Cassell, London.*

Moss, R. (1991) *Europe Animal Welfare Concern and Chaos.* UFAW, Potters Bar.

Nuffield Council on Bioethics (2005) *The Ethics of Research Involving Animals* (report). London.

OECD (1982) *GLP in the Testing of Chemicals,* Final Report of the OECD Expert Group on GLP. Organisation for Economic Cooperation and Development, Geneva.

Orlans, B. (1993) *In the Name of Science – Issues of Responsible Animal Experimentation.* Oxford University Press, New York.

Paton, W. (1984) *Man and Mouse.* Oxford University Press, Oxford.

PCD Circulars (2000–2006) Letters to Certificate Holders containing topical information on A(SP)A matters. Home Office, London.

Phillips, M.T. & Sechzer, J.A. (1989) *Animal Research and Ethical Conflict. An Analysis of the Scientific Literature.* Springer-Verlag, Berlin.

Poole, T. (1997) Happy animals make good science. *Laboratory Animals* 31: 116–24.

Radford, Mike (2001) *Animal Welfare Law in Britain.* Oxford University Press, Oxford.

RCVS (1992) *Code of Practice for Named Veterinary Surgeon employed in Scientific Procedure Establishments and Breeding and Supplying Establishments under the Animals (Scientific Procedures) Act 1986.* Royal College of Veterinary Surgeons, London.

RCVS (1999) *Legislation Affecting the Veterinary Profession in the UK.* Royal College of Veterinary Surgeons, London.

Revision of Directive 86/609/EEC, Report of Sub-Group (2003). European Commission.

Rollins, B. (1989) *The Unheeded Cry.* Oxford University Press, Oxford.

RSPCA (1994) *Ethical Concern for Animals.* Royal Society for the Prevention of Cruelty to Animals, Horsham.

RSPCA (1998) *Progressing the Ethical Review Process.* RSPCA, Horsham.

RSPCA (2005) *Resource Book for Lay Members of ERPs.* RSPCA, Horsham.

Russell, W.M.S. and Burch, R.L. (1992) *The Principles of Humane Experimental Technique.* UFAW, South Mimms.

Ryder, Richard D. (1975) *Victims of Science.* Davis-Poynter, London.

Sainsbury, D. (1991) *Farm Animal Welfare: Cattle, Pigs and Poultry.* Blackwell Science, Oxford.

Sandys-Wynch, G. (1984) *Animal Law.* Shaw and Sons, London.

Seamer, J.H. and Wood, M. (eds) (1999) *Safety in the Animal House,* 2nd edn. Laboratory Animal Handbooks No. 13. Laboratory Animals Ltd, London.

Short, D. & Woodnott, D. (1978) *The IAT Manual of Laboratory Animal Practice and Techniques.* Granada Publishing Ltd, London.

Singer, P. (1992) *Applied Ethics.* Oxford University Press, Oxford.

Smith, J.A. & Boyd, K.M. (1991) *Lives in the Balance.* Oxford University Press, Oxford.

Smith, M.W. (ed) (1984) *Report of the Working Party on Courses for Animal Licencees. Laboratory Animals* 18: 209–20.

Smyth, D.H. (1978) *Alternatives to Animal Experimentation.* Scolar Press, Aldershot.

Tester, K. (1992) *Animals and Society.* Routledge, London.

UFAW (ed T.B. Poole) (1999) *Handbook on the Care and Management of Laboratory Animals,* 7th edn. Blackwell Science, Oxford.

United Kingdom Coordinating Committee on Cancer Research (UK CCCR) (1988) *Guidelines for the Welfare of Animals in Experimental Neoplasia.* UK CCCR, London.

Wards Journal of Refinement Recognition (1997) Refinement Project Manuscript Summaries. Wards Inc., Vienna.

Wilkins, David B. (ed) (1997) *Animal Welfare in Europe, European Legislation and Concerns.* Kluwer Law International, London.

Table of Cases

Table of Statutes

To some readers there may appear to be gaps in the above list. Early Acts such as the Cruelty to Animals Act 1876 may be relevant to the subject and are referred to in the text. They are, however, no longer applicable, having been repealed. Some Acts dealing with animals, such as the Performing Animal (Regulation) Act 1925, are hardly relevant to the law on laboratory animals. The Breeding and Sale of Dogs (Welfare) Act 1999 for example, is concerned with the pet trade so does not apply to Designated Establishments. What has been said about this list is equally applicable to the following lists of Statutory Instruments and European Directives.

Table of Statutory Instruments

Statutory Instruments specific to Northern Ireland, Scotland or Wales, associated with the above Statutory Instruments, where appropriate, are on the same page.

Variation of this legislation may also occur in the Isle of Man and the Channel Isles. For example, A(SP)A does not apply to the Isle of Man but covers British owned ships within 12 miles territorial waters limit (cf. Inspectorate Annual Report 2005, p. 18.)

Table of European Legislation

European Directives

European Regulations

Index